# The Super Easy

## Keto Air Fryer Cookbook

*1500 Days of Tasty Air Fryer Creations for Carb-Conscious Foodies to Take Your Keto Journey to New Heights | Full Color Edition*

**Felicia W. McCloud**

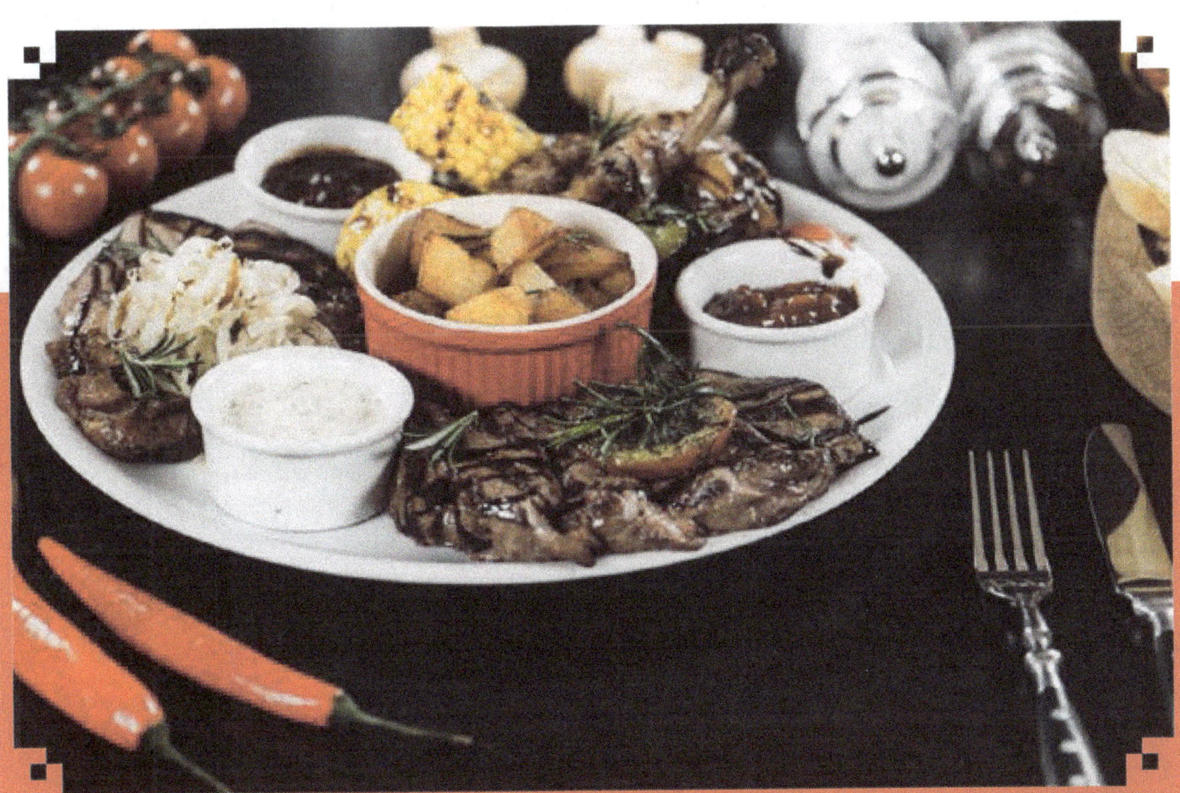

**Manufactured in:** USA

**Cover Art:** DANIELLE REES

**Production Editor:** SIENNA ADAMS

**Production Manager:** SARAH JOHNSON

**Interior Design:** DANIELLE REES

**Art Producer:** BROOKE WHITE

**Editor:** AALIYAH LYONS

**Photography:** MICHAEL SMITH

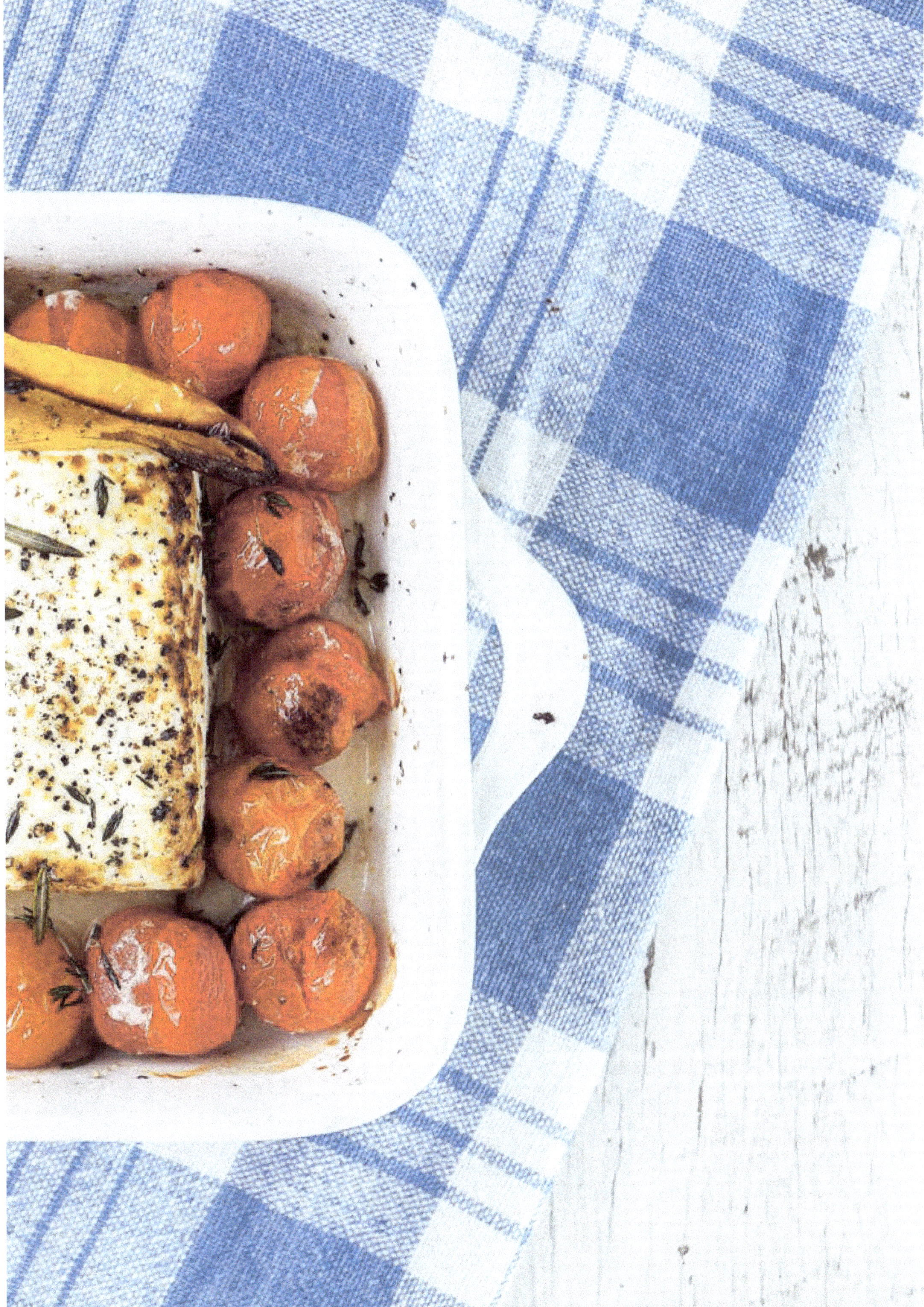

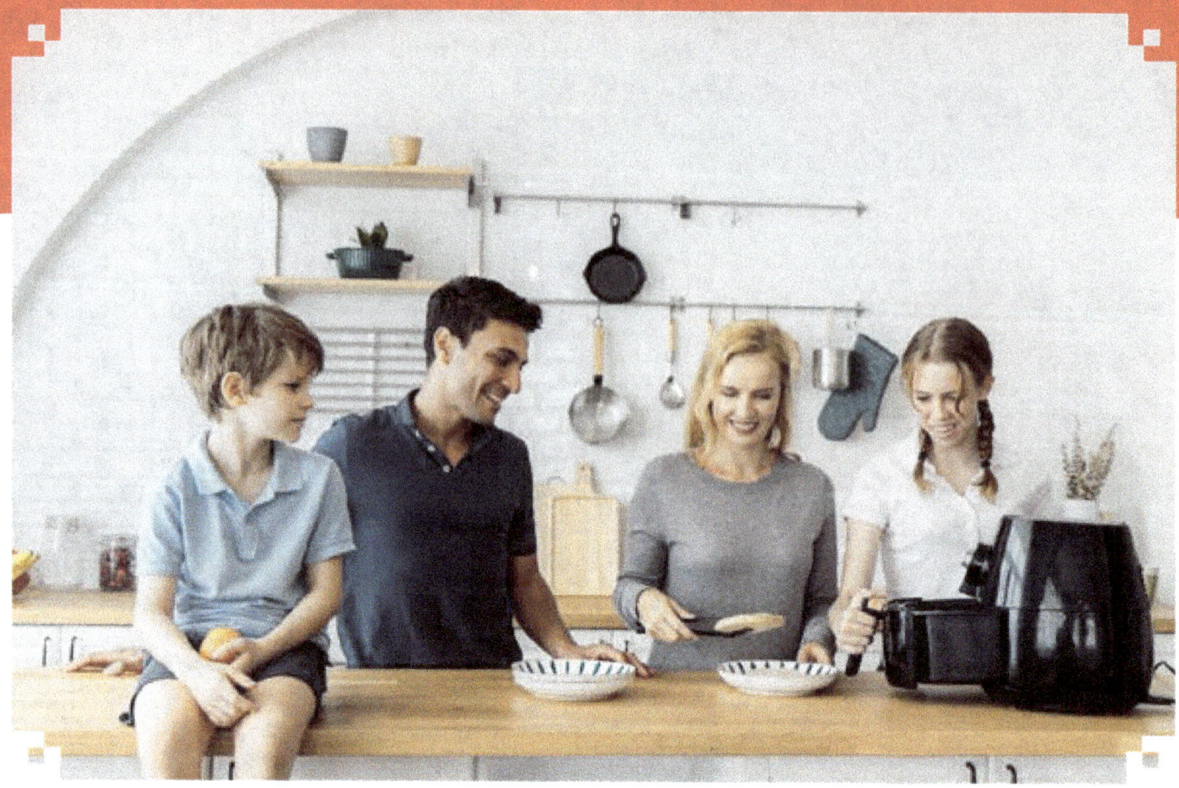

# Table Of Contents

# Introduction

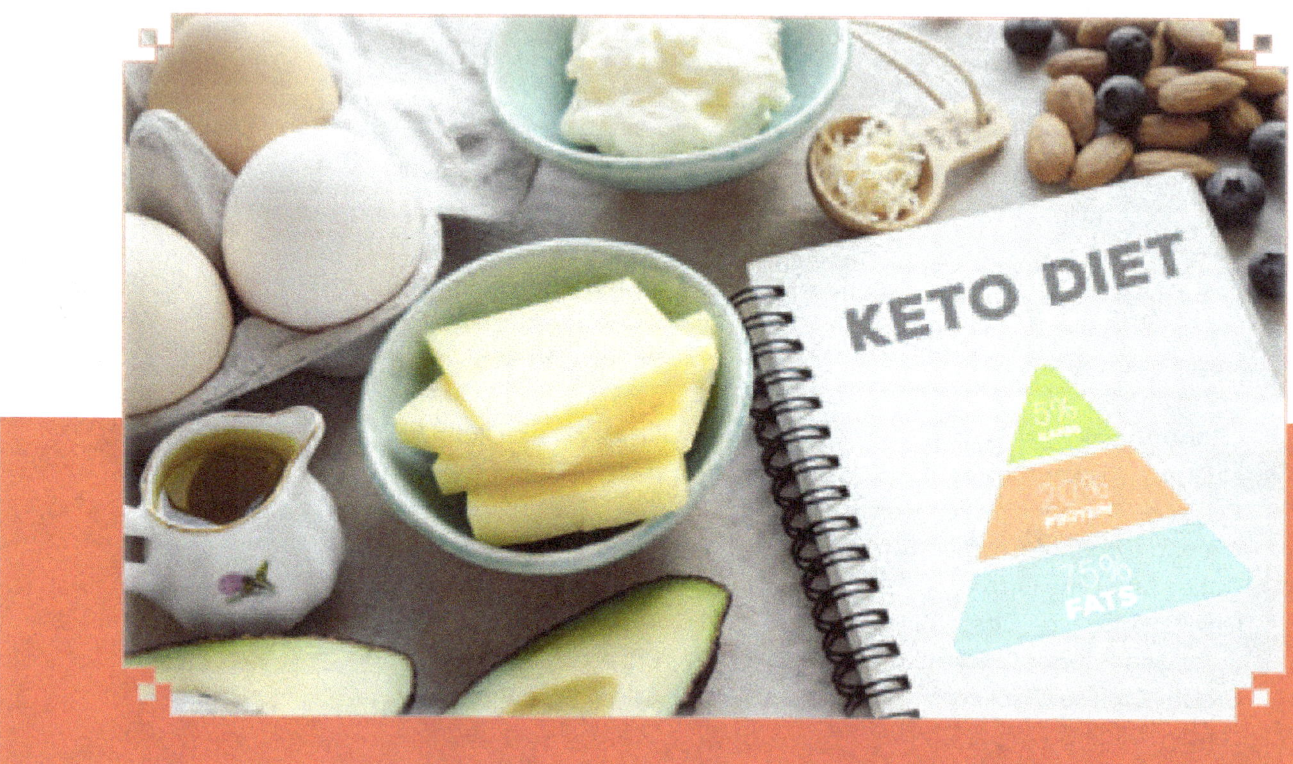


*Just a few years back, if you had told me my kitchen would evolve to exist without a deep fryer and a pantry bursting at the seams with carbs, I would have chuckled and brushed off the notion. Back then, cooking was my ticket to indulgence—an immersive sensory journey often drenched in sweetness and rich fats. Fast forward to today, and I stand as a proud flag-bearer of the ketogenic lifestyle, with my air fryer gleaming under the spotlight on my countertop. This isn't just the story of how my cooking habits did a 180; it's the tale of my personal transformation, a journey of self-discovery wrapped up in altering my diet.*

*My bond with food has always been a rollercoaster ride. Childhood memories are laden with heartwarming, lavish meals, though not always the epitome of nutritional wisdom. As a young adult, convenience often won the battle over health, spiraling into a pattern of not-so-great eating habits. It wasn't until my body began to protest, hinting at the toll these choices were taking, that I paused to reflect. That moment of realization was my first step towards what would unfold as the most enriching expedition of my life.*

*Stumbling upon the ketogenic diet felt like discovering a new continent. Initially, I met the idea with skepticism—cutting out almost all carbs seemed like an uphill battle. Yet, as I peeled back the layers of keto's scientific foundation and listened to countless success stories, curiosity got the better of me, and I decided to dive in. Transitioning was anything but easy. Battling cravings, weathering the storm of initial lethargy, and climbing the steep learning curve of tweaking my cooking repertoire were daunting challenges. But my resolve was steel.*

*The air fryer—a thoughtful gift from my husband, Justin—initially gathered dust, a foreign intruder in my culinary sanctuary. Yet, as I began to experiment with keto-friendly recipes, I saw the light. This gadget transformed into an indispensable ally, enabling me to relish the crispy, savory delights I missed, sans the guilt traditionally associated with fried foods. This epiphany was a game-changer.*

*Sharing my keto air fryer marvels on social media, I was taken aback by the avalanche of responses. Individuals from diverse backgrounds reached out, eager for guidance, sharing their journeys, and seeking advice. It struck me how my personal saga struck a chord with many on a quest for a healthier life, without forgoing the pleasures of eating. This burgeoning sense of community propelled me to keep pushing the envelope, to keep sharing, and above all, to never stop learning.*

*Compiling a cookbook had never crossed my mind, yet it emerged as a heartfelt extension of my keto voyage. Putting together my recipes and musings felt like I was handing over a piece of my soul to the world. It's a tribute to my evolution from a keto skeptic to a fervent advocate of mindful, delectable cooking with the air fryer.*

*To those embarking on their own keto adventure, my advice is simple: patience is a virtue, embrace experimentation, and cherish the journey. The road to a healthier lifestyle is a personal one, but it's dotted with the joys of discovery and self-care. Through sharing my story, my culinary creations, and my insights, I aim to light the way for others on their path to wellness and contentment.*

## Dedication

*To Justin, my unwavering beacon in the uncharted waters of a flourless kitchen and the eye of the storm in our oil-less culinary escapades. Your steadfast faith in the transformative power of a single kitchen gadget and a simple diet overhaul became the bedrock of our joint quest for a vibrant, healthful existence. This journey, peppered with the sizzle of the air fryer and laughter echoing in our carb-conscious kitchen, is a testament to our partnership. It's a celebration of the flavorsome, nutritious meals we've crafted, not just from the ingredients we've mixed but from the love and camaraderie that fills our home. This book is a homage to every experiment you've taste-tested, every word of encouragement, and our shared culinary adventures. May our keto kitchen inspire as much joy in others as you have in me.*

# Chapter 1

## Kick Off Your Keto Journey with An Air Fryer

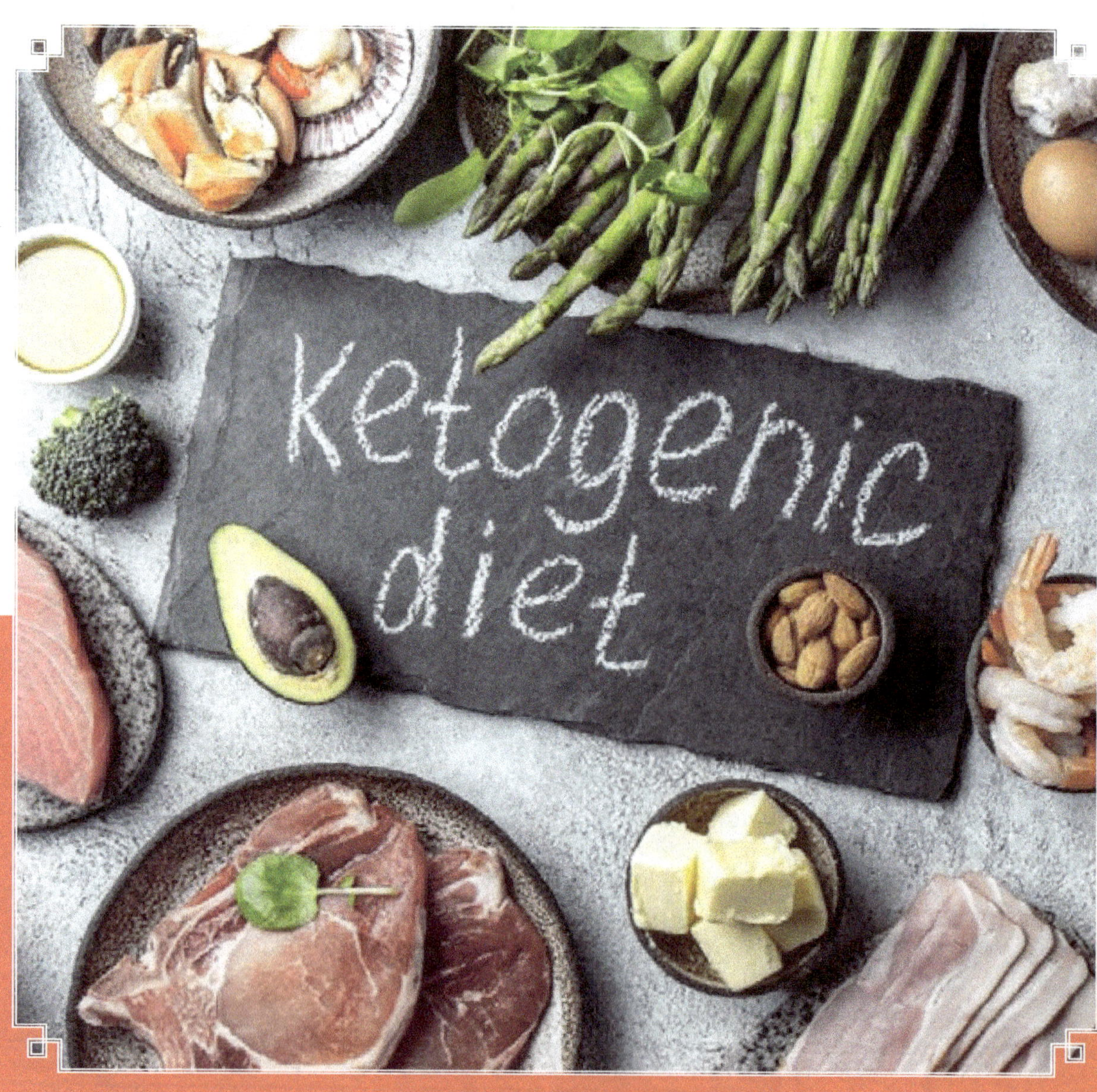

# Understanding Keto

Imagine a diet that not only helps shed pounds but also powers up your brain. Welcome to the ketogenic diet, a revolutionary approach to eating that's reshaping bodies and minds. This low-carbohydrate, high-fat regimen pushes your body into ketosis, a metabolic state where fat, instead of carbs, becomes your main energy source. This transition not only facilitates weight loss but also leads to a decrease in blood sugar and insulin levels, potentially improving various health markers.

The ketogenic diet traces its roots back to the 1920s, initially devised as a therapeutic diet for epilepsy patients. From its medical origins, the keto diet has evolved, becoming a popular lifestyle choice for those looking to tackle a range of health challenges beyond seizure control. Its versatility and effectiveness in managing conditions such as diabetes, Alzheimer's disease, and certain cancers have added to its acclaim, transforming it from a niche medical solution to a global health trend.

The debate around the ketogenic diet is fueled by contrasting opinions, especially concerning its high fat content. Critics worry about the possible implications for heart health, citing increased cholesterol risks. However, proponents, bolstered by studies, argue that many individuals following keto experience improved cholesterol levels, showcasing the diet's potential for cardiovascular benefits.

**ADHERING TO THE KETOGENIC DIET MEANS EMBRACING FOODS LIKE:**

- Meats and fish
- Butter and eggs
- Cheese and heavy cream
- Oils and nuts
- Avocados and seeds
- Low-carb vegetables

**CONVERSELY, IT INVOLVES AVOIDING:**

- Sugary foods and grains
- Starches and fruits
- Beans and legumes
- Root vegetables
- Low-fat or diet products

Before embarking on the ketogenic journey, consulting with a healthcare professional is advisable to ensure it aligns with your health goals and needs. Through careful planning and informed choices, the ketogenic diet can be a transformative tool for body and mind.

- Benefits of Keto Diet

The ketogenic diet, with its unique approach to nutritional intake, offers a myriad of benefits that extend beyond simple weight loss, making it a favored dietary choice for many. At the heart of these advantages is the diet's ability to induce ketosis, a state where the body efficiently burns fat for fuel, leading to several impactful health outcomes.

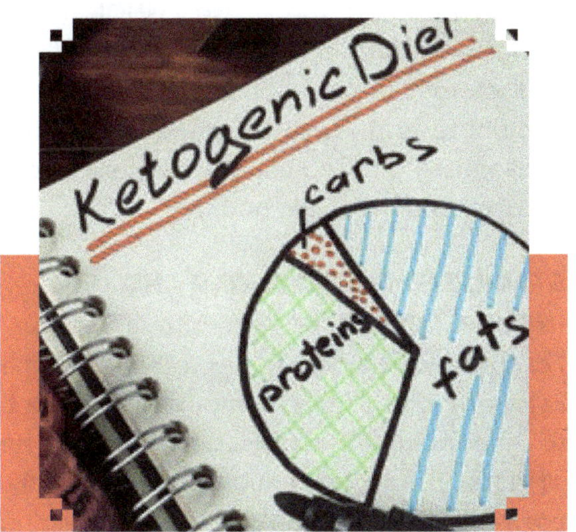

## WEIGHT LOSS ACCELERATION

The keto diet's high-fat, low-carbohydrate regime is instrumental in promoting rapid weight loss. By reducing carb intake, the body is forced to turn to its fat stores for energy, a process that leads to more effective weight reduction compared to traditional low-fat diets. The diet's ability to stabilize blood sugar levels further aids in managing and preventing cravings, making it easier for individuals to adhere to their dietary plans.

## ENHANCED BRAIN FUNCTION

A standout benefit of the ketogenic diet is its positive impact on brain health. Ketones, produced during ketosis, are a more efficient fuel source for the brain than glucose. This shift in energy supply can lead to improved cognitive functions, such as enhanced memory, focus, and clarity. Additionally, the diet has been linked to a reduced risk of neurological disorders, offering a preventive strategy against conditions like Alzheimer's and Parkinson's disease.

## IMPROVED HEART HEALTH

Despite concerns over its high-fat content, the keto diet can improve heart health by positively influencing cholesterol levels. By increasing the intake of healthy fats, many individuals see a rise in HDL (good cholesterol) and a decrease in LDL (bad cholesterol) levels. These changes can contribute to a lower risk of heart disease, challenging the traditional views on dietary fat and cardiovascular health.

## STABILIZED BLOOD SUGAR AND INSULIN LEVELS

For those with diabetes or prediabetes, the ketogenic diet offers a compelling approach to managing blood sugar levels. The significant reduction in carbohydrate intake prevents large spikes in blood sugar, helping to maintain more stable levels throughout the day. This stability can not only aid in diabetes management but also reduce the risk of developing type 2 diabetes.

## INCREASED ENERGY AND IMPROVED PHYSICAL PERFORMANCE

Many adherents of the keto diet report a sustained increase in energy levels and an improvement in physical performance. The constant fuel supply provided by ketones avoids the energy dips associated with fluctuating blood sugar levels, enabling more consistent energy availability for physical activities.

# Mastering the Keto Lifestyle

Mastering the ketogenic lifestyle is a journey that goes beyond merely adopting a new way of eating; it's about embracing a comprehensive approach to health and well-being that requires dedication, adaptation, and a bit of creativity. Here are key strategies to thrive on this transformative path:

## EDUCATION IS KEY

Understanding the science behind ketosis and how different foods affect your body is crucial. Educate yourself about the nutritional content of foods, the importance of maintaining electrolyte balance, and how to interpret signs from your body. Knowledge empowers you to make informed decisions and navigate challenges.

## PLANNING AND PREPARATION

Success with keto often comes down to planning. Prepare your meals in advance to avoid the temptation of off-plan eating. Stock your pantry with keto-friendly staples, and consider meal prepping to save time during busy weeks. This preparation extends to social situations; having keto-friendly options available can help maintain your lifestyle choices without feeling isolated.

## CUSTOMIZATION FOR SUSTAINABILITY

The keto diet isn't one-size-fits-all. Tailor the diet to fit your lifestyle, preferences, and health goals. Some may thrive on a strict ketogenic plan, while others may find success with a more flexible approach. Listen to your body and adjust your macronutrient intake to find what works best for you, ensuring long-term adherence and satisfaction.

## COMMUNITY AND SUPPORT

Embarking on a keto journey can be challenging, but you don't have to do it alone. Engage with the keto community, whether online or in-person. Sharing experiences, recipes, and tips can provide motivation and support. Family and friends can also offer encouragement, so communicate your goals and how they can support you.

## MINDFUL EATING AND LIFESTYLE CHANGES

Adopting a mindful approach to eating, focusing on the quality of foods and the enjoyment of meals, can enhance your keto experience. Additionally, integrating regular physical activity that you enjoy can boost your health benefits and support your mental well-being.

## PATIENCE AND FLEXIBILITY

Transitioning to a keto lifestyle may come with its set of challenges, including the initial adaptation phase commonly known as the "keto flu." Be patient with your body as it adjusts to burning fat for fuel. Recognize and celebrate your progress, no matter how small, and be flexible to make changes as needed.

## CONTINUOUS LEARNING AND ADAPTATION

The keto landscape is always evolving, with new research, recipes, and resources becoming available. Stay curious and open to learning. Adapting your approach based on new insights can keep the diet exciting and maintain your engagement over time.

# Introducing the Air Fryer

Introducing the air fryer, a revolutionary kitchen appliance that has transformed the way we cook and enjoy our favorite foods. This compact device, celebrated for its efficiency and versatility, uses rapid air technology to mimic the results of deep frying, giving you that coveted crispy texture without the excessive use of oil. It's a game-changer for health-conscious food lovers and busy home cooks alike, offering a healthier alternative to traditional frying methods while significantly cutting down cooking time.

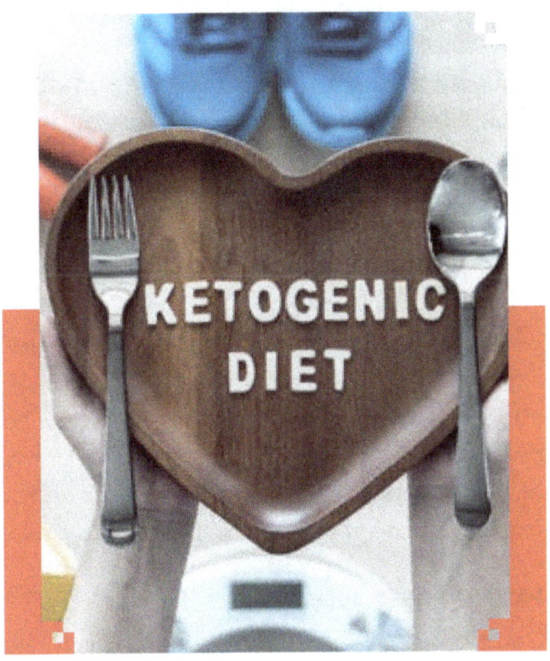

• How Air Fryers Work

The air fryer works by circulating hot air around the food placed in its basket, cooking it quickly and evenly from all angles. This process results in a crispy outer layer while keeping the inside tender and juicy, mirroring the taste and texture of deep-fried foods but with a fraction of the fat and calories. The appeal of the air fryer doesn't stop at frying; it's a multi-functional powerhouse capable of grilling, roasting, and baking, making it a versatile addition to any kitchen.

• Advantages of Air Frying for Keto

**EASE OF USE AND CONVENIENCE**

One of the air fryer's biggest selling points is its simplicity. With straightforward settings and a hassle-free cleanup process—thanks to its non-stick, dishwasher-safe parts—cooking with an air fryer is a breeze. Its compact size makes it ideal for kitchens of all sizes, from spacious homes to small apartments.

**HEALTHIER COOKING**

By using significantly less oil, the air fryer provides a healthier way to enjoy fried foods, reducing the risk of heart disease and other health issues associated with high-fat diets. It's an excellent tool for those looking to improve their diet without sacrificing the joy of eating.

**VERSATILITY**

Beyond frying, the air fryer's capabilities extend to roasting vegetables, baking cookies, and even grilling meats to perfection. Its ability to cook a wide variety of dishes makes it a valuable appliance for experimenting with new recipes and cuisines.

**ENERGY EFFICIENCY**

Compared to conventional ovens, air fryers heat up quickly and cook food faster, saving time and energy. This efficiency is not only good for the environment but also helps lower utility bills.

• Maintenance and Care Tips

1. Cool Down: Always allow the air fryer to cool completely before attempting to clean or maintain it.
2. Disassemble: Remove the basket, tray, or any removable parts from the air fryer.
3. Wash Removable Parts: Clean the basket, tray, and any other removable components with warm, soapy water. Most of these parts are dishwasher safe for convenience.
4. Wipe the Exterior: Use a damp cloth to gently wipe the exterior of the air fryer.
5. Interior Cleaning: Clean the interior with a soft, non-abrasive sponge or cloth to remove grease or food particles. Avoid harsh chemicals or scouring pads that could damage the surface.
6. Check the Heating Element: Regularly inspect the heating element for any food particles or debris and carefully remove them.
7. Dry Thoroughly: Ensure all parts are completely dry before reassembling and storing the air fryer.
8. Store Properly: Keep the air fryer in a dry, cool place when not in use to prevent any damage or wear.

# Air Fryer Cooking Techniques

Air fryer cooking techniques harness the appliance's unique rapid air technology to produce delicious, healthier versions of traditionally fried favorites, along with an array of other dishes. Mastering these techniques can elevate your cooking, allowing you to fully explore the air fryer's versatility. Here are some essential tips and methods to enhance your air frying experience:

## PREHEATING FOR PERFECTION

Much like a traditional oven, preheating your air fryer can lead to better cooking results. A preheated air fryer ensures that food starts cooking immediately upon basket entry, promoting an even, crispy finish. Most models require just a few minutes to reach the desired temperature, making this a quick step not to be skipped.

## BASKET MANAGEMENT FOR EVEN COOKING

To achieve that perfectly even, crispy texture, avoid overcrowding the basket. Air circulation is crucial in air frying, and overcrowding impedes this process, leading to unevenly cooked food. Cooking in batches might take a bit more time but will deliver superior results. For some foods, shaking the basket halfway through the cooking time or flipping them over can also encourage an even cook.

## OIL USAGE

While one of the air fryer's appeals is reduced oil usage, a light spritz of oil on food can enhance its texture, contributing to a more desirable crispy finish. Use an oil sprayer for a light, even coat. Opt for oils with a high smoke point, such as avocado or light olive oil, to prevent smoking.

## BREADING

For breaded items, ensure your breading process is thorough. Lightly pressing the coating onto your food helps it stick better during the cooking process. Pre-toasting panko breadcrumbs can add an extra level of crunchiness to your finished dish.

## TEMPERATURES AND TIMING

Understanding that cooking times and temperatures can vary significantly from traditional frying or baking is key. Start with the recommended settings in recipes but be prepared to adjust. Due to the air fryer's efficient design, cooking times are often shorter, so it's wise to check on your dish periodically to prevent overcooking.

## ACCESSORIES AND TOOLS

Utilizing air fryer accessories can expand your cooking options. From baking pans to racks, these tools can help you bake, grill, or layer food more effectively within the air fryer. Silicone or parchment liners can also make cleanup even easier while preventing sticking.

## CREATIVE COOKING BEYOND FRYING

Embrace the air fryer's potential beyond just frying. Experiment with roasting vegetables for a charred, smoky flavor, baking moist cakes, or even "hard-boiling" eggs. The air fryer's ability to cook quickly with minimal oil opens the door to endless culinary experimentation.

The ketogenic diet, renowned for its health benefits and weight loss potential, emphasizes low-carb, high-fat foods that transform the body into a fat-burning machine. When paired with the innovative cooking technology of the air fryer, achieving your keto goals becomes both effortless and enjoyable. This dynamic duo allows for the creation of delicious, crispy meals that adhere to keto guidelines without sacrificing flavor or texture. As we venture into the realm of keto-friendly recipes, the air fryer stands as an invaluable tool, enabling us to explore a variety of dishes that are not only healthy but also incredibly satisfying. Let's dive into the recipes that will tantalize your taste buds while keeping you firmly on the path to ketosis.

# Chapter 2

## 4-Week Meal Plan

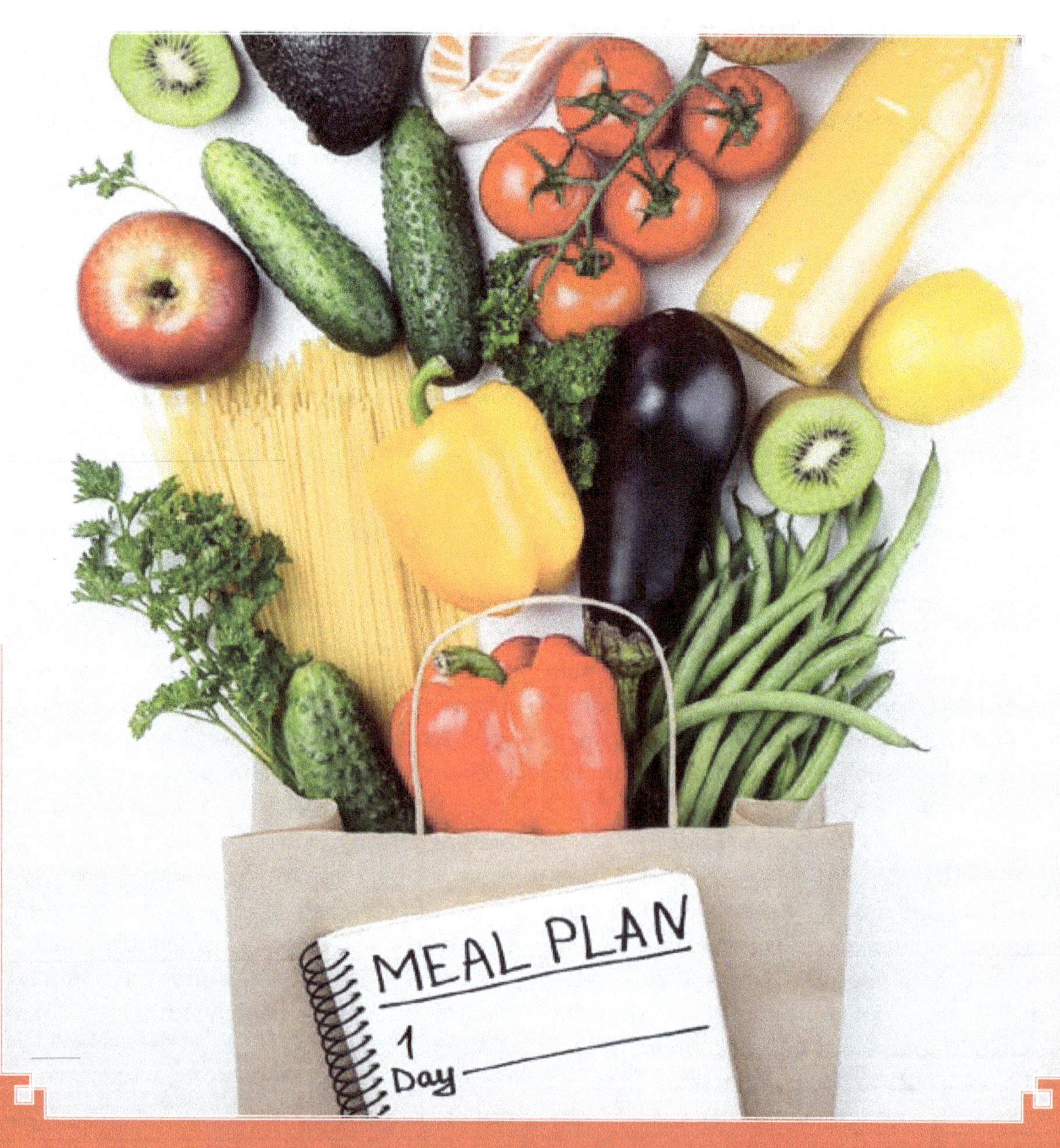

# Week 1

**DAY 1:**
- Breakfast: Coconut Veggie and Eggs Bake
- Lunch: Almond Coconut Chicken Tenders
- Snack: Italian Eggplant Bites
- Dinner: Sweet and Spicy Spare Ribs

Total for the day:
**Calories: 1091; Fat: 64.5 g; Fiber: 15.9 g;Carbs: 26.1 g; Protein: 68.7 g**

**DAY 2:**
- Breakfast: Coconut Veggie and Eggs Bake
- Lunch: Almond Coconut Chicken Tenders
- Snack: Italian Eggplant Bites
- Dinner: Sweet and Spicy Spare Ribs

Total for the day:
**Calories: 1091; Fat: 64.5 g; Fiber: 15.9 g;Carbs: 26.1 g; Protein: 68.7 g**

**DAY 3:**
- Breakfast: Coconut Veggie and Eggs Bake
- Lunch: Almond Coconut Chicken Tenders
- Snack: Italian Eggplant Bites
- Dinner: Sweet and Spicy Spare Ribs

Total for the day:
**Calories: 1091; Fat: 64.5 g; Fiber: 15.9 g;Carbs: 26.1 g; Protein: 68.7 g**

**DAY 4:**
- Breakfast: Coconut Veggie and Eggs Bake
- Lunch: Almond Coconut Chicken Tenders
- Snack: Italian Eggplant Bites
- Dinner: Sweet and Spicy Spare Ribs

Total for the day:
**Calories: 1091; Fat: 64.5 g; Fiber: 15.9 g;Carbs: 26.1 g; Protein: 68.7 g**

**DAY 5:**
- Breakfast: Coconut Veggie and Eggs Bake
- Lunch: Sweet and Spicy Spare Ribs
- Snack: Italian Eggplant Bites
- Dinner: Cilantro Cod Mix

Total for the day:
**Calories: 1089; Fat: 63.5 g; Fiber: 13.9 g; Carbs: 25.1 g; Protein: 64.7 g**

**DAY 6:**
- Breakfast: Coconut Veggie and Eggs Bake
- Lunch: Sweet and Spicy Spare Ribs
- Snack: Savory Herb Cloud Eggs
- Dinner: Cilantro Cod Mix

Total for the day:
**Calories: 1078; Fat: 67 g; Fiber: 6 g; Carbs: 12 g; Protein: 63 g**

**DAY 7:**
- Breakfast: Southwestern Breakfast Taco
- Lunch: Cilantro Cod Mix
- Snack: Savory Herb Cloud Eggs
- Dinner: Cilantro Cod Mix

Total for the day:
**Calories: 1164; Fat: 72 g; Fiber: 9 g; Carbs: 22 g; Protein: 62 g**

# Week 2

**DAY 1:**
- Breakfast: Cheddar Tomatoes Hash
- Lunch: Lemon-Dijon Boneless Chicken
- Snack: Seafood Balls
- Dinner: Roasted Cilantro Lamb Chops

Total for the day:
**Calories: 1009; Fat: 51.4 g; Fiber: 9 g; Carbs: 14.9 g; Protein: 73.6 g**

**DAY 2:**
- Breakfast: Cheddar Tomatoes Hash
- Lunch: Lemon-Dijon Boneless Chicken
- Snack: Seafood Balls

- Dinner: Roasted Cilantro Lamb Chops

Total for the day:
**Calories: 1009; Fat: 51.4 g; Fiber: 9 g; Carbs: 14.9 g; Protein: 73.6 g**

## DAY 3:

- Breakfast: Cheddar Tomatoes Hash
- Lunch: Lemon-Dijon Boneless Chicken
- Snack: Seafood Balls
- Dinner: Roasted Cilantro Lamb Chops

Total for the day:
**Calories: 1009; Fat: 51.4 g; Fiber: 9 g; Carbs: 14.9 g; Protein: 73.6 g**

## DAY 4:

- Breakfast: Cheddar Tomatoes Hash
- Lunch: Lemon-Dijon Boneless Chicken
- Snack: Seafood Balls
- Dinner: Roasted Cilantro Lamb Chops

Total for the day:
**Calories: 1009; Fat: 51.4 g; Fiber: 9 g; Carbs: 14.9 g; Protein: 73.6 g**

## DAY 5:

- Breakfast: Fried Bacon
- Lunch: Lemon-Dijon Boneless Chicken
- Snack: Dry Rub Chicken Wings
- Dinner: Roasted Cilantro Lamb Chops

Total for the day:
**Calories: 1347; Fat: 85.4 g; Fiber: 5.1 g; Carbs: 9.4 g; Protein: 108.7 g**

## DAY 6:

- Breakfast: Fried Bacon
- Lunch: Lemon-Dijon Boneless Chicken
- Snack: Dry Rub Chicken Wings
- Dinner: Roasted Cilantro Lamb Chops

Total for the day:
**Calories: 1347; Fat: 85.4 g; Fiber: 5.1 g; Carbs: 9.4 g; Protein: 108.7 g**

## DAY 7:

- Breakfast: Fried Bacon
- Lunch: Fijan Coconut Fish
- Snack: Dry Rub Chicken Wings
- Dinner: Fijan Coconut Fish

Total for the day:
**Calories: 1679; Fat: 101.4 g; Fiber: 7.9 g; Carbs: 21.2 g; Protein: 170.1 g**

# Week 3

## DAY 1:

- Breakfast: Kale Omelet
- Lunch: Cream Cheese Chicken
- Snack: Garlic Endives and Scallions
- Dinner: Pork and Spinach Stew

Total for the day:
**Calories: 880; Fat: 31.1 g; Fiber: 9.4 g; Carbs: 13.9 g; Protein: 59.1 g**

## DAY 2:

- Breakfast: Kale Omelet
- Lunch: Cream Cheese Chicken
- Snack: Garlic Endives and Scallions
- Dinner: Pork and Spinach Stew

Total for the day:
**Calories: 880; Fat: 31.1 g; Fiber: 9.4 g; Carbs: 13.9 g; Protein: 59.1 g**

## DAY 3:

- Breakfast: Kale Omelet
- Lunch: Cream Cheese Chicken
- Snack: Garlic Endives and Scallions
- Dinner: Pork and Spinach Stew

Total for the day:
**Calories: 880; Fat: 31.1 g; Fiber: 9.4 g; Carbs: 13.9 g; Protein: 59.1 g**

**DAY 4:**
- Breakfast: Kale Omelet
- Lunch: Cream Cheese Chicken
- Snack: Garlic Endives and Scallions
- Dinner: Pork and Spinach Stew

Total for the day:
**Calories: 880; Fat: 31.1 g; Fiber: 9.4 g; Carbs: 13.9 g; Protein: 59.1 g**

**DAY 5:**
- Breakfast: Butter Donuts
- Lunch: Cream Cheese Chicken
- Snack: Balsamic Cabbage Mix
- Dinner: BBQ Skirt Steak

Total for the day:
**Calories: 799; Fat: 36.9 g; Fiber: 7.4 g; Carbs: 11.5 g; Protein: 92.8 g**

**DAY 6:**
- Breakfast: Butter Donuts
- Lunch: BBQ Skirt Steak
- Snack: Balsamic Cabbage Mix
- Dinner: BBQ Skirt Steak

Total for the day:
**Calories: 1035; Fat: 53.8 g; Fiber: 8 g; Carbs: 12.3 g; Protein: 113.7 g**

**DAY 7:**
- Breakfast: Butter Donuts
- Lunch: BBQ Skirt Steak
- Snack: Balsamic Cabbage Mix
- Dinner: BBQ Skirt Steak

Total for the day:
**Calories: 1035; Fat: 53.8 g; Fiber: 8 g; Carbs: 12.3 g; Protein: 113.7 g**

# Week 4

### DAY 1:
- Breakfast: Cod and Shallot Frittata
- Lunch: Jalapeño Popper Chicken
- Snack: Walnut and Rum Cookies
- Dinner: Caraway Seeds Lamb Loin

Total for the day:
**Calories: 1182; Fat: 72.1 g; Fiber: 4.5 g; Carbs: 12.5 g; Protein: 116.6 g**

### DAY 2:
- Breakfast: Cod and Shallot Frittata
- Lunch: Jalapeño Popper Chicken
- Snack: Walnut and Rum Cookies
- Dinner: Caraway Seeds Lamb Loin

Total for the day:
**Calories: 1182; Fat: 72.1 g; Fiber: 4.5 g; Carbs: 12.5 g; Protein: 116.6 g**

### DAY 3:
- Breakfast: Cod and Shallot Frittata
- Lunch: Jalapeño Popper Chicken
- Snack: Walnut and Rum Cookies
- Dinner: Caraway Seeds Lamb Loin

Total for the day:
**Calories: 1182; Fat: 72.1 g; Fiber: 4.5 g; Carbs: 12.5 g; Protein: 116.6 g**

### DAY 4:
- Breakfast: Breakfast Eggs with Swiss Chard and Ham
- Lunch: Jalapeño Popper Chicken
- Snack: Walnut and Rum Cookies
- Dinner: Caraway Seeds Lamb Loin

Total for the day:
**Calories: 1383;Fat: 80.9 g; Fiber: 5.4 g; Carbs: 10.3 g;Protein: 153.2 g**

### DAY 5:
- Breakfast: Breakfast Eggs with Swiss Chard and Ham
- Lunch: Jalapeño Popper Chicken
- Snack: Walnut and Rum Cookies

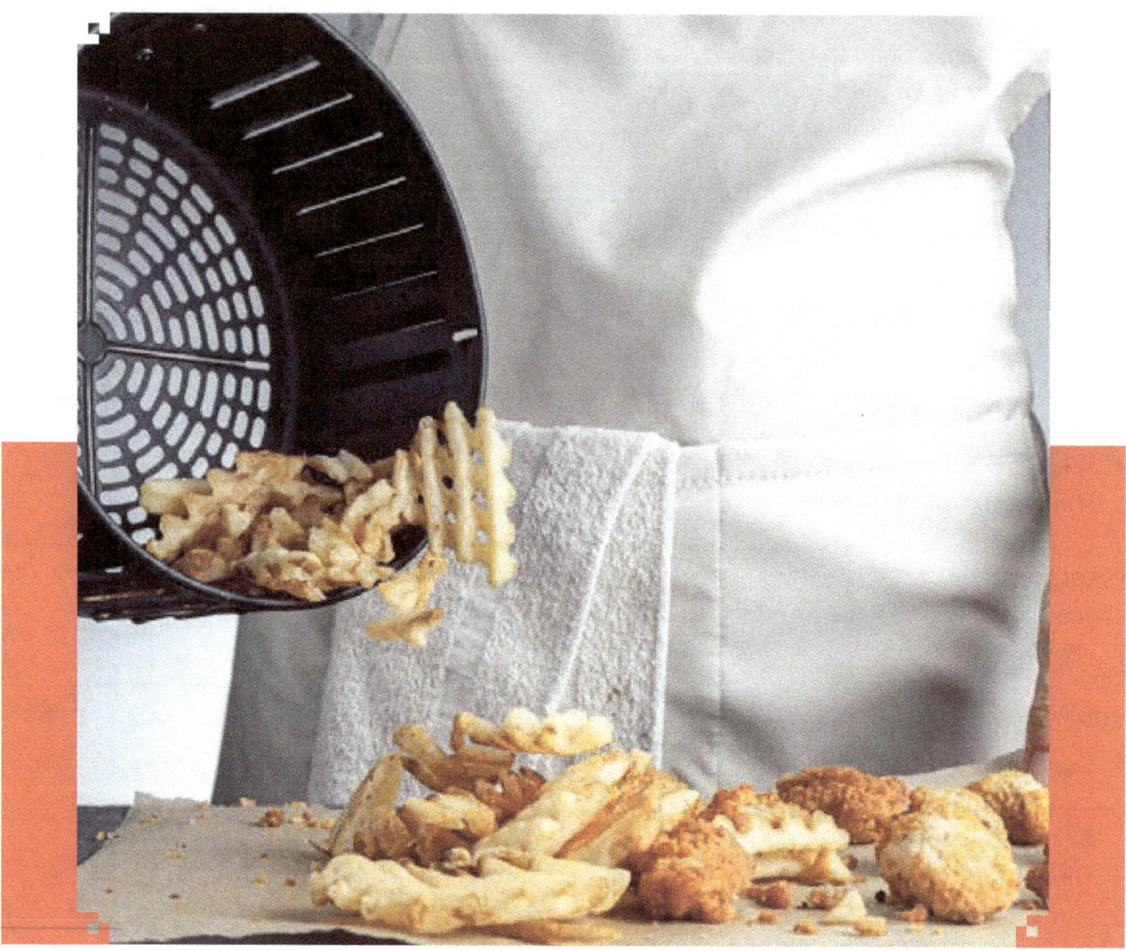

* Dinner: Crispy Green Beans

Total for the day:
**Calories: 1383;Fat: 80.9 g; Fiber: 5.4 g; Carbs: 10.3 g;Protein: 153.2 g**

### DAY 6:
* Breakfast: Breakfast Eggs with Swiss Chard and Ham
* Lunch: Jalapeño Popper Chicken
* Snack: Walnut and Rum Cookies
* Dinner: Crispy Green Beans

Total for the day:

**Calories: 1383;Fat: 80.9 g; Fiber: 5.4 g; Carbs: 10.3 g;Protein: 153.2 g**

### DAY 7:
* Breakfast: Breakfast Eggs with Swiss Chard and Ham
* Lunch: Jalapeño Popper Chicken
* Snack: Walnut and Rum Cookies
* Dinner: Crispy Green Beans

Total for the day:
**Calories: 1383;Fat: 80.9 g; Fiber: 5.4 g; Carbs: 10.3 g;Protein: 153.2 g**

# Chapter 3

## Appetizers and Desserts

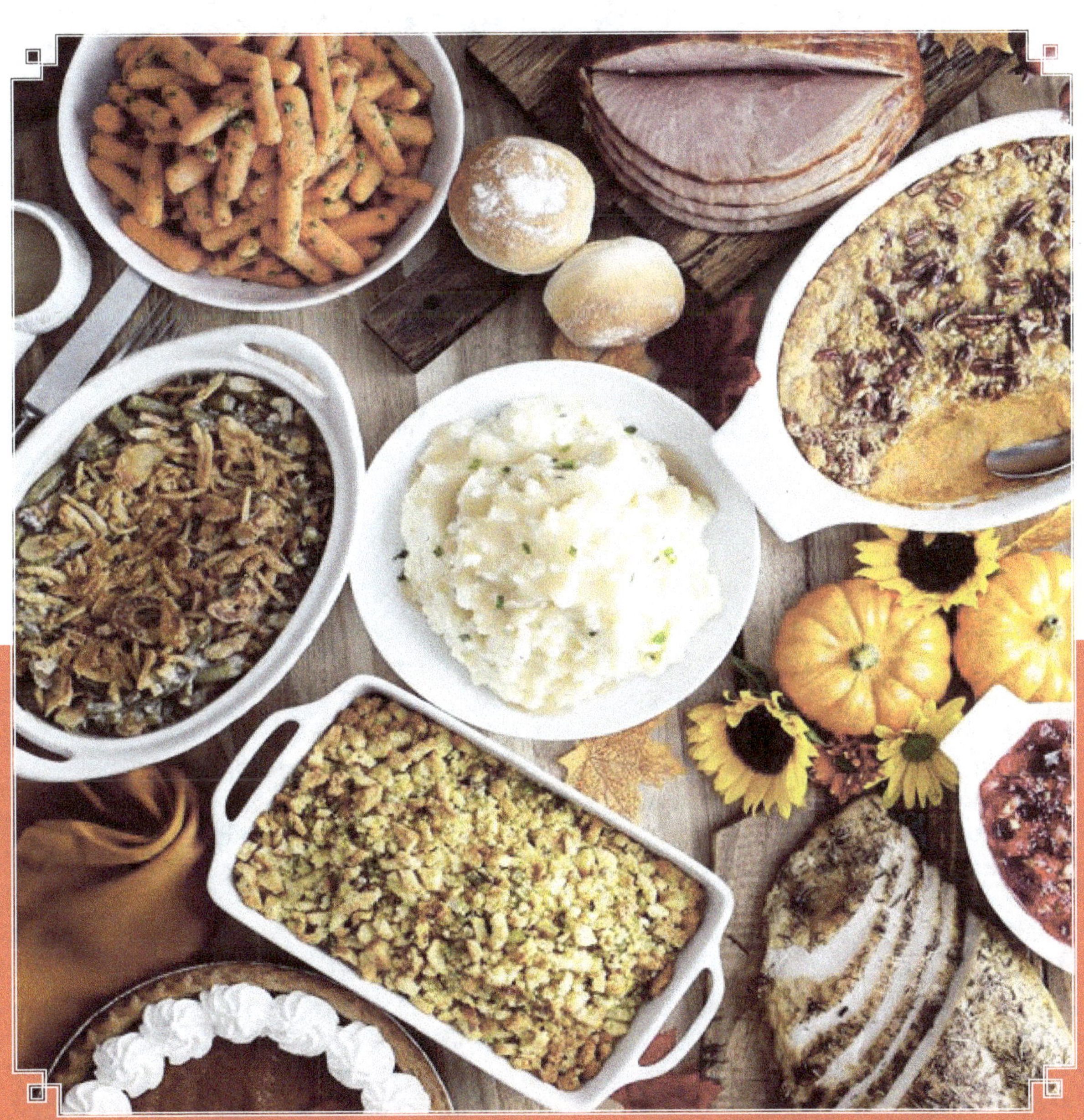

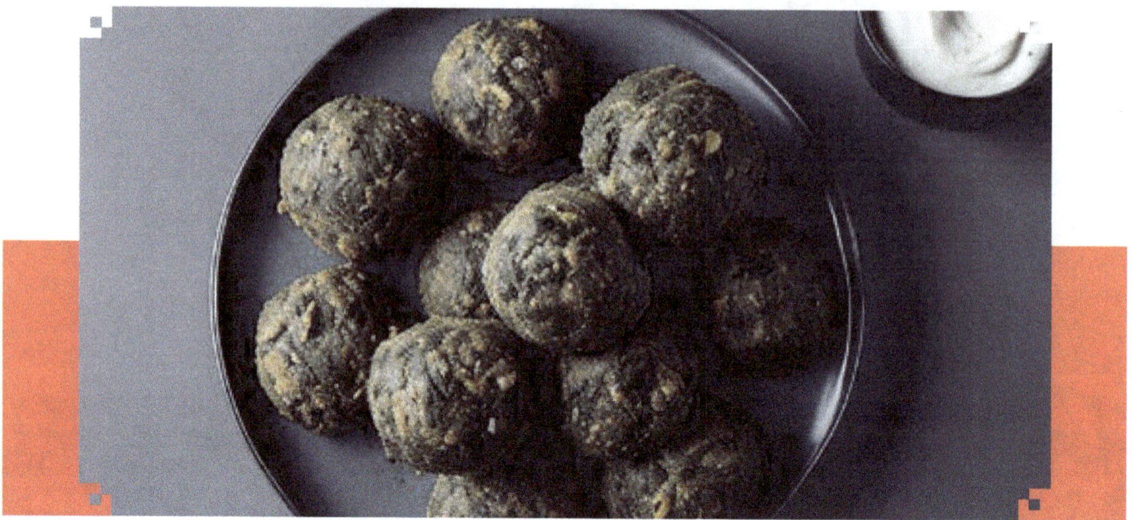

## Greek Calamari Appetizer

**Prep time: 10 minutes | Cook time: 20 minutes |
Serves 6**

- 1 ½ pounds calamari tubes, cleaned, cut into rings
- Sea salt and ground black pepper, to taste
- 2 tablespoons lemon juice
- 1/2 cup almond meal
- 2 eggs, whisked
- 1/4 cup buttermilk

1. Preheat your Air Fryer to 390 °F. Rinse the calamari and pat it dry. Season with salt and black pepper. Drizzle lemon juice all over the calamari.
2. Arrange them in the Air Fryer cooking basket. Spritz with cooking oil and cook for 9 to 12 minutes, shaking the basket occasionally. Work in batches.
3. Serve with toothpicks. Bon appétit!

**PER SERVING**

Calories: 254 | Fat: 15.8g | Carbs: 2.6g |
Protein: 25.3g |Fiber: 0.1g

## Cheese Balls with Spinach

**Prep time: 10 minutes | Cook time: 15 minutes |
Serves 4**

- 1/4 cup milk
- 2 eggs
- 1 cup cheese
- 2 cups spinach, torn into pieces
- 1/3 cup flaxseed meal
- 1/2 teaspoon baking powder
- 2 tablespoons canola oil
- Salt and ground black pepper, to taste

1. Add all the ingredients to a food processor or blender; then, puree the ingredients until it becomes dough.
2. Next, roll the dough into small balls. Preheat your air fryer to 310 °F.
3. Cook the balls in your Air Fryer for about 12 minutes or until they are crispy. Bon appétit!

**PER SERVING**

Calories: 314 | Fat: 24.1g | Carbs: 5.7g | Protein:
11.3g |Fiber: 4.1g

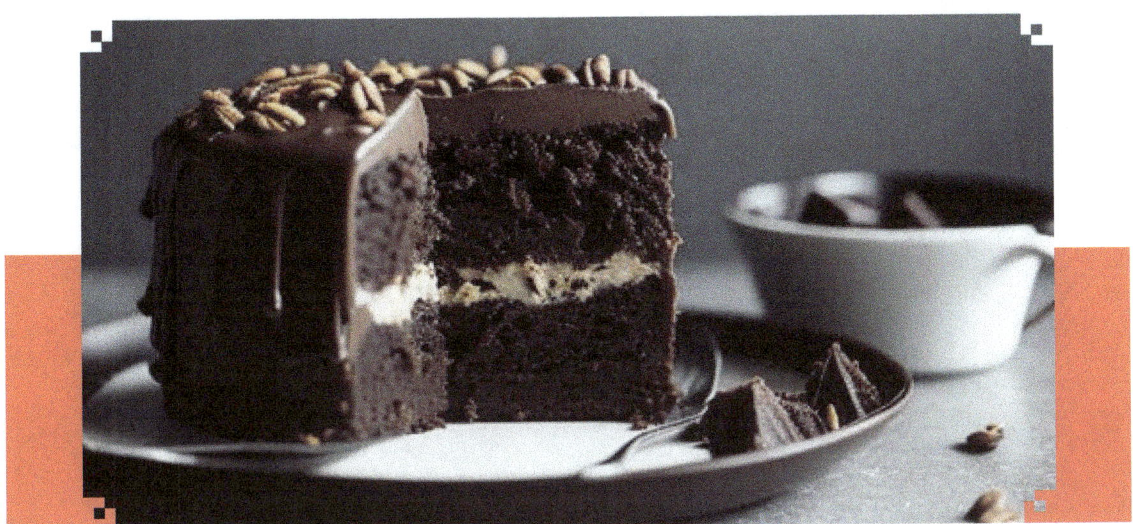

## Pumpkin Pie-Spiced Pork Rinds

**Prep time: 5 minutes | Cook time: 5 minutes | Serves 4**

- 3 ounces plain pork rinds
- 2 tablespoons salted butter, melted
- 1 teaspoon pumpkin pie spice
- ¼ cup confectioners' erythritol

1. In a large bowl, toss pork rinds in butter. Sprinkle with pumpkin pie spice, then toss to evenly coat.
2. Place pork rinds into ungreased air fryer basket. Adjust the temperature to 400°F and set the timer for 5 minutes. Pork rinds will be golden when done.
3. Transfer rinds to a medium serving bowl and sprinkle with erythritol. Serve immediately.

**PER SERVING**

Calories: 173 | Protein: 12g | Fiber: 0g | Carbs: 0g | Fat: 13g

## Fudge Cake with Pecans

**Prep time: 10 minutes | Cook time: 30 minutes | Serves 6**

- 1/2 cup butter, melted
- 1/2 cup swerve
- 1 teaspoon vanilla essence
- 1/2 cup almond flour
- 1/2 teaspoon baking powder
- 1 ounce bakers' chocolate, unsweetened
- 1/4 cup pecans, finely chopped

1. Start by preheating your Air Fryer to 350 °F. Now, lightly grease six silicone molds.
2. In a mixing dish, beat the melted butter with the swerve until fluffy. Next, stir in the vanilla and egg and beat again.
3. Fold in the chocolate and pecans; mix to combine. Bake in the preheated Air Fryer for 20 to 22 minutes. Enjoy!

**PER SERVING**

Calories: 253 | Fat: 25.5g | Carbs: 6.4g | Protein: 4.2g | Fiber: 3.4g

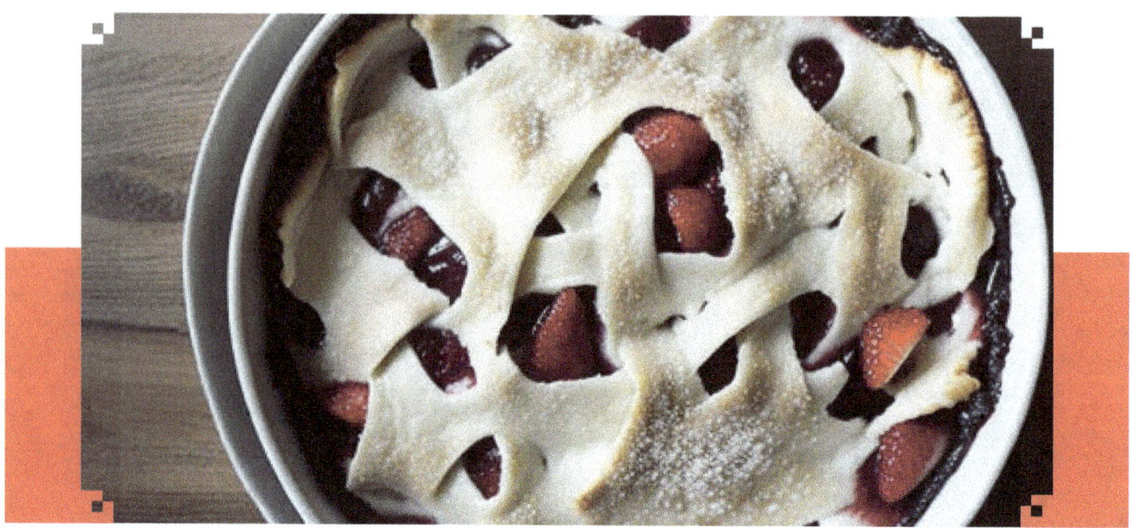

## Must-Serve Thai Prawns

**Prep time: 10 minutes | Cook time: 10 minutes | Serves 4**

- 16 prawns, cleaned and deveined
- 1 medium-sized egg, whisked
- 1 tablespoon curry powder
- 1/2 teaspoon grated fresh ginger
- 1/2 cup coconut flour

1. Toss the prawns with salt, pepper, cumin powder, and lemon juice.
2. In a mixing dish, place the whisked egg, beer, baking powder, curry, and the ginger; mix to combine well.
3. In another mixing dish, place the coconut flour.
4. Air-fry at 360 °F for 5 minutes; turn them over, press the power button again and cook for additional 2 to 3 minutes. Bon appétit!

**PER SERVING**

Calories: 259 | Fat: 15.8g | Carbs: 3.4g | Protein: 4.1g | Fiber: 1.8g

## Berry Pie

**Prep time: 5 minutes |Cook time: 20 minutes |Serves 8**

- 5 egg whites
- 1/3 cup swerve
- 1 and ½ cups almond flour
- Zest of 1 lemon, grated
- 1/3 cup butter, melted
- 2 cups strawberries, sliced
- Cooking spray

1. In a bowl, whisk egg whites well. Add the rest of the ingredients except the cooking spray gradually and whisk everything.
2. Grease a tart pan with the cooking spray, and pour the strawberries mix. Put the pan in the air fryer and cook at 370 °F for 20 minutes.
3. Cool down, slice and serve.

**PER SERVING**

Calories: 182g |Fat: 12g |Fiber: 1g |Carbs: 6g |Protein: 5 g

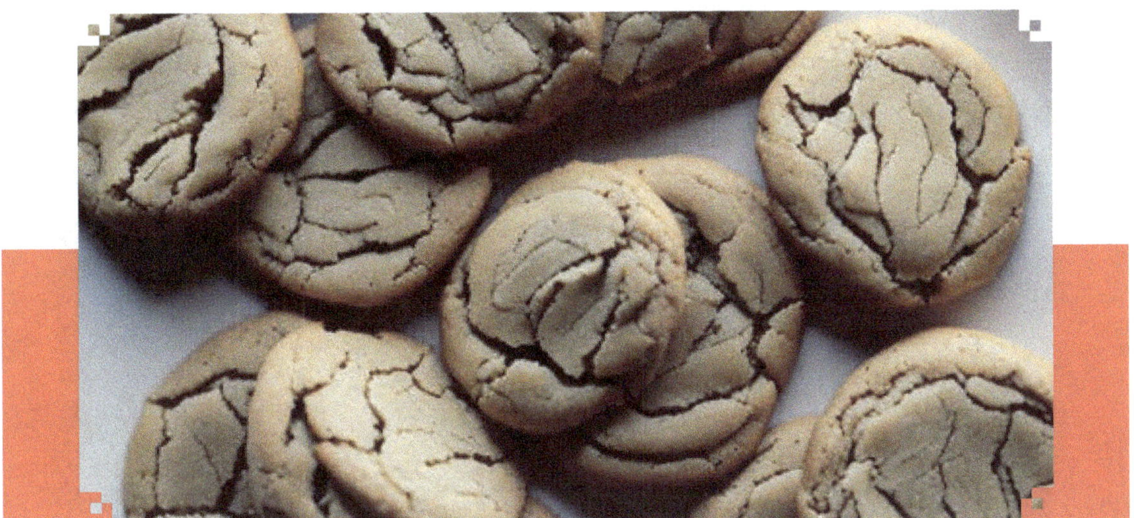

## 15-Minute Orange Galettes

**Prep time: 10 minutes | Cook time: 15 minutes | Serves 6**

- 1 cup almond meal
- 1/2 cup coconut flour
- 3 eggs
- 1⁄3 cup milk
- 2 tablespoons monk fruit
- 1 ½ teaspoons baking powder
- 3 tablespoons orange juice
- A pinch of turmeric

1. Grab two mixing bowls. Combine dry ingredients in the first bowl.
2. In the second bowl, combine all wet ingredients. Add wet mixture to the dry mixture and mix until smooth and uniform.
3. Air-fry for 4 to 5 minutes at 345 °F. Work in batches. Dust with confectioners' swerve if desired. Bon appétit!

**PER SERVING**

Calories: 177 | Fat: 13.5g | Carbs: 7.3g | Protein: 7.4g | Fiber: 2.6g

## Walnut and Rum Cookies

**Prep time: 10 minutes | Cook time: 40 minutes | Serves 8**

- 1/2 cup walnuts, ground
- 1/2 cup coconut flour
- 1 cup almond flour
- 3/4 cup swerve
- 2 tablespoons rum
- 1/2 teaspoon pure vanilla extract
- 1/2 teaspoon pure almond extract

1. In a mixing dish, beat the butter with swerve, vanilla, and almond extract until light and fluffy. Then, throw in the flour and ground walnuts; add in rum.
2. Roll the dough into small cookies and place them on the Air Fryer cake pan; gently press each cookie using a spoon.
3. Bake butter cookies for 15 minutes in the preheated Air Fryer. Bon appétit!

**PER SERVING**

Calories: 228 | Fat: 22.3g | Carbs: 4g | Protein: 3.5g | Fiber: 2.3g

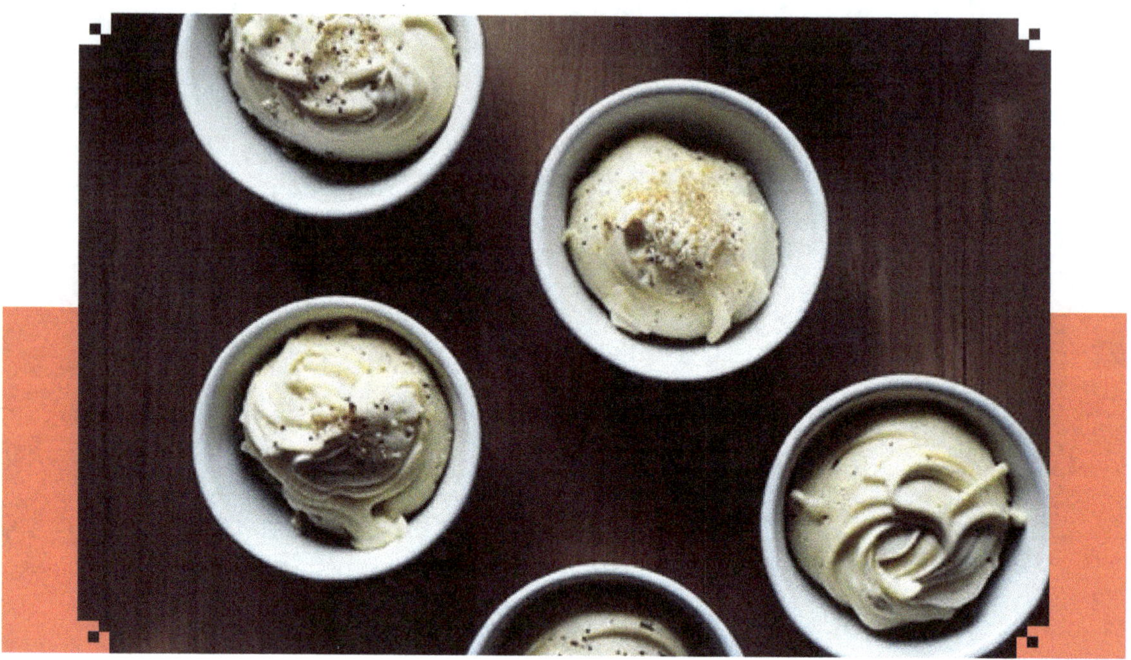

## Easy Spanish Churros

**Prep time: 10 minutes | Cook time: 20 minutes | Serves 4**

- 3/4 cup water
- 1 tablespoon swerve
- 1/4 teaspoon sea salt
- 3/4 cup almond flour
- 2 eggs

1. To make the dough, boil the water in a the swerve, salt, nutmeg, and cloves; cook until dissolved.
2. Remove from the heat; fold in the eggs one at a time, stirring to combine well.
3. Cook at 410 °F for 6 minutes, working in batches. Bon appétit!

**PER SERVING**

Calories: 321 | Fat: 31.1g | Carbs: 4.4g | Protein: 8.4g | Fiber: 2.3g

## Cream Cups

**Prep time: 5 minutes |Cook time: 10 minutes |Serves 6**

- 2 tablespoons butter, melted
- 8 ounces cream cheese, soft
- 3 tablespoons coconut, shredded and unsweetened
- 3 eggs
- 4 tablespoons swerve

1. In a bowl, mix all the ingredients and whisk really well.
2. Divide into small ramekins, put them in the fryer and cook at 320 °F and bake for 10 minutes.
3. Serve cold.

**PER SERVING**

Calories: 164g| Fat: 4g| Fiber: 2g| Carbs: 5g| Protein: 5g

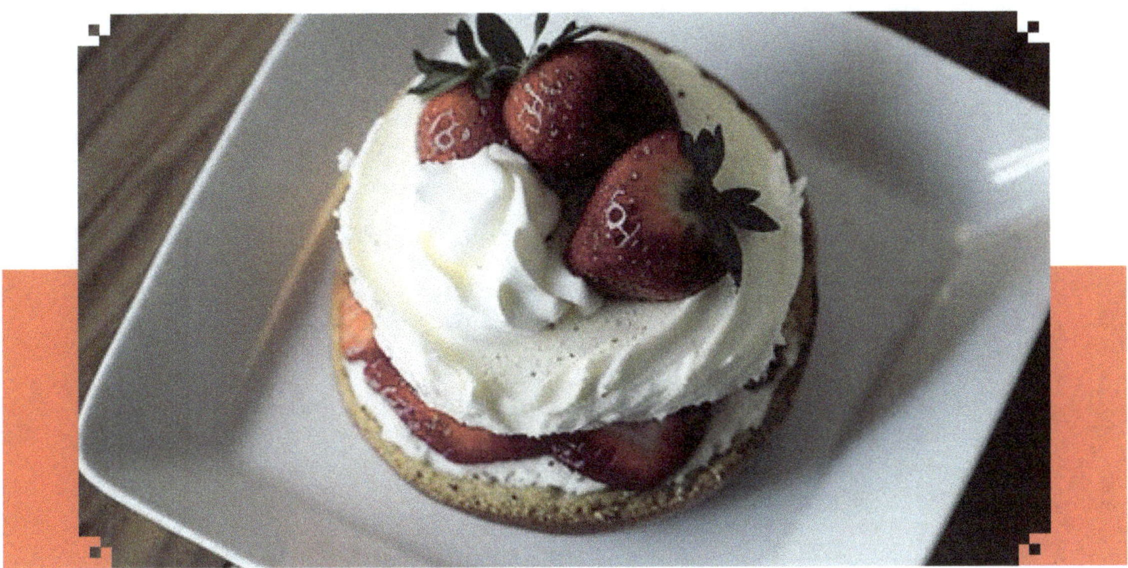

# Chocolate Doughnut Holes

**Prep time: 10 minutes | Cook time: 6 minutes | Makes 20 doughnut holes**

- 1 cup blanched finely ground almond flour
- ½ cup low-carb vanilla protein powder
- ½ cup granular erythritol
- ¼ cup unsweetened cocoa powder
- ½ teaspoon baking powder
- 2 large eggs, whisked
- ½ teaspoon vanilla extract

1. Mix all ingredients in a large bowl until a soft dough forms. Separate and roll dough into twenty balls, about 2 tablespoons each.
2. Doughnut holes will be golden and firm when done. Let cool completely before serving, about 10 minutes.

**PER SERVING**

Calories: 103 | Protein: 8g | Fiber: 2g | Carbs: 8g | Fat: 7g

# Strawberry Shortcake

**Prep time: 1 hour 10 minutes | Cook time: 25 minutes | Serves 6**

- 2 tablespoons coconut oil
- 1 cup blanched finely ground almond flour
- 2 large eggs, whisked
- ½ cup granular erythritol
- 1 teaspoon baking powder

1. In a large bowl, combine coconut oil, flour, eggs, erythritol, baking powder, and vanilla. Pour batter into an ungreased 6" round nonstick baking dish.
2. Remove dish from fryer and let cool 1 hour.
3. Once cooled, top cake with whipped cream and strawberries to serve.

**PER SERVING**

Calories: 235 | Protein: 6g | Fiber: 2g | Carbs: 3g | Fat: 21g

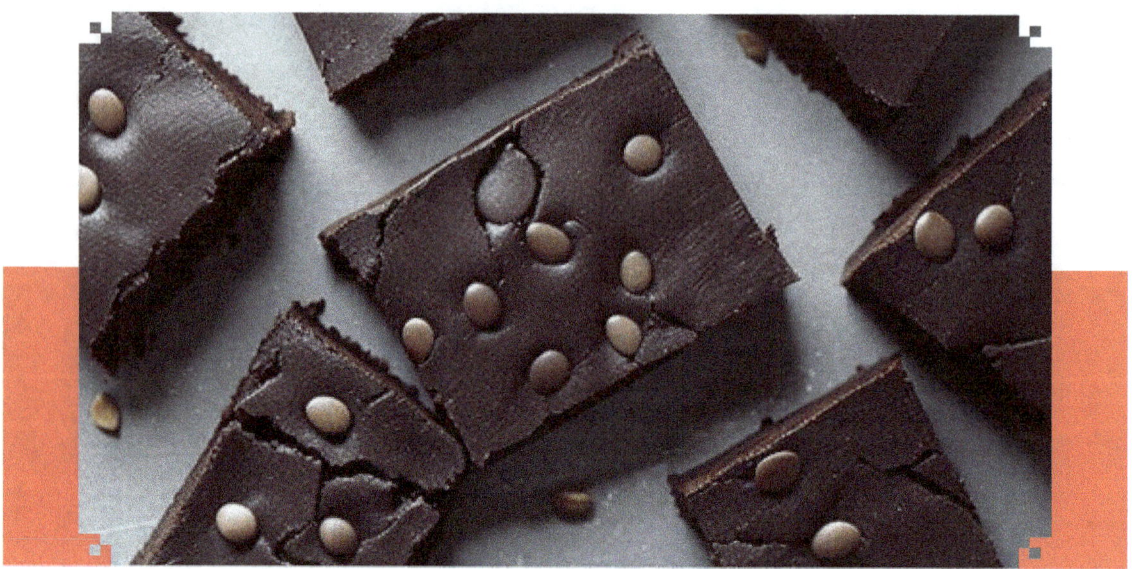

## Cream Cheese Shortbread Cookies

**Prep time: 40 minutes | Cook time: 20 minutes | Makes 12 cookies**

- ¼ cup coconut oil, melted
- 2 ounces cream cheese, softened
- ½ cup granular erythritol
- 1 large egg, whisked
- 1 teaspoon almond extract

1. Combine all ingredients in a large bowl to form a firm ball.
2. Place dough on a sheet of plastic wrap and roll into a 12"-long log shape. Roll log in plastic wrap and place in refrigerator 30 minutes to chill.
3. Let cool 15 minutes before serving to avoid crumbling.

**PER SERVING**

Calories: 175 | Protein: 5g | Fiber: 2g | Carbs: 2g | Fat: 16g

## Double Chocolate Brownies

**Prep time: 15 minutes | Cook time: 25 minutes | Serves 8**

- 1 cup almond flour
- ½ cup unsweetened cocoa powder
- ½ teaspoon baking powder
- 1 teaspoon vanilla extract
- 2 tablespoons mini semisweet chocolate chips

1. Preheat the air fryer to 350°F. Line an 8-inch cake pan with parchment paper and brush with vegetable oil.
2. Air fry for 15 to 20 minutes until the edges are set. (The center should still appear slightly undercooked.) Let cool completely before slicing. To store, up to 3 days.

**PER SERVING**

Calories: 230 | Protein: 8g | Carbs: 10g | Fat: 20g | Fiber: 3g

# Chapter 4

## Breakfasts

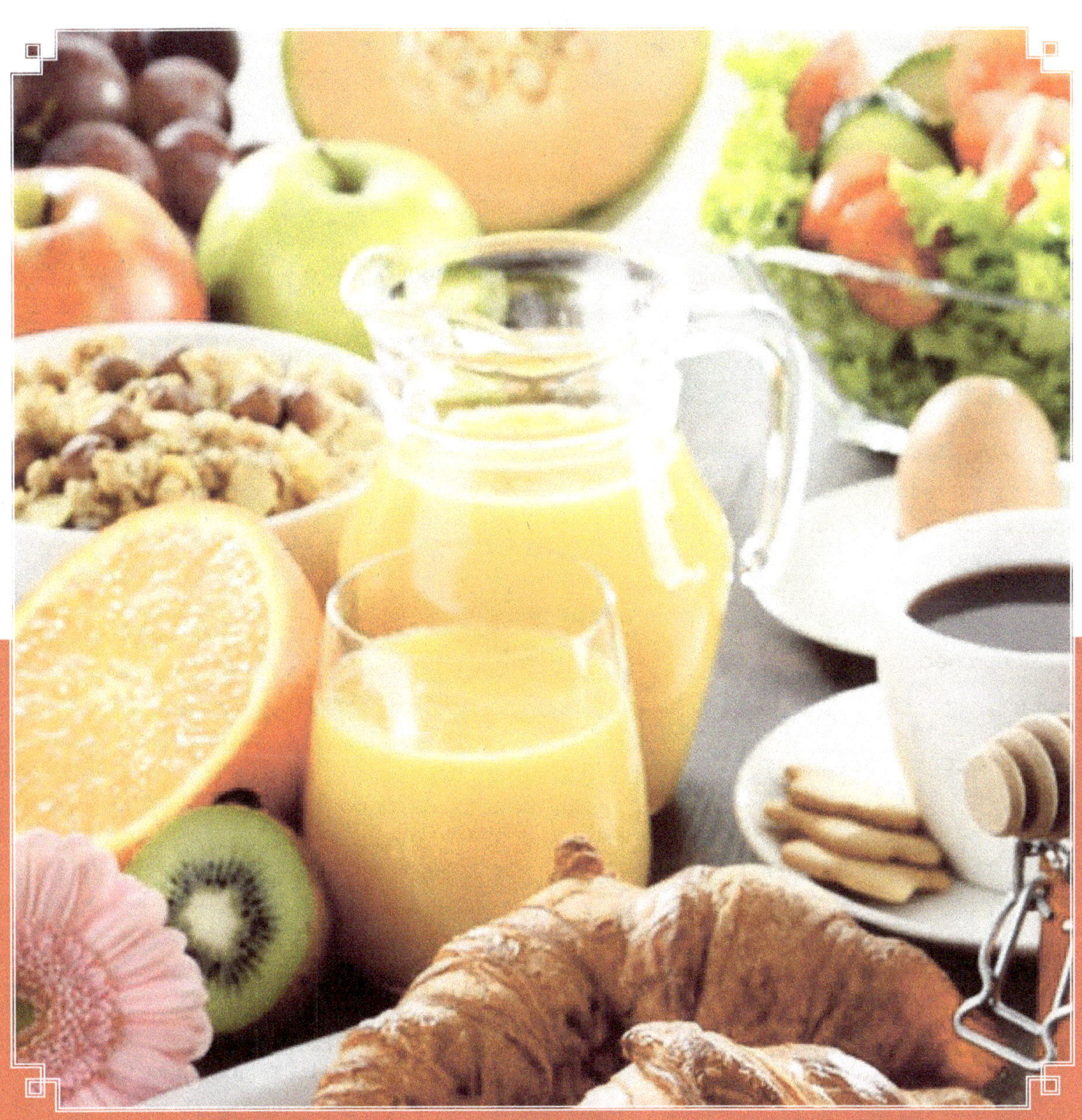

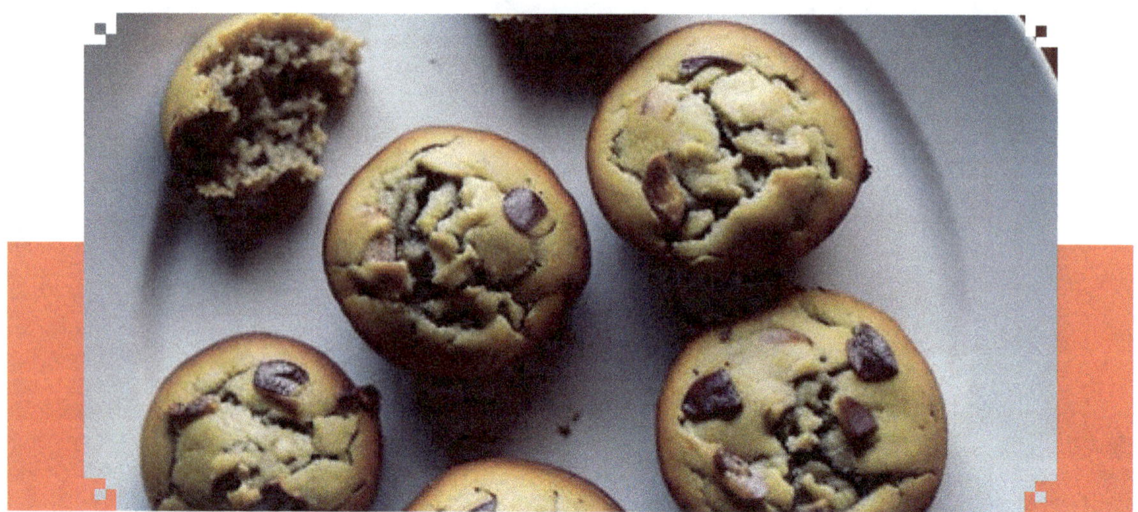

# Coconut Veggie and Eggs Bake

**Prep time: 5 minutes |Cook time: 30 minutes |Serves 6**

- cooking spray
- 2 spring onions, chopped
- 1 teaspoon thyme, chopped
- salt and black pepper to the taste
- 1 cup coconut cream
- 4 eggs, whisked
- 1 cup cheddar cheese, grated

1. In a bowl, mix all the ingredients except the cooking spray and the cheese and whisk well.
2. Grease a pan that fits the air fryer put the pan in the machine and cook at 350 °F for 30 minutes.
3. Divide between plates and serve for breakfast.

**PER SERVING**

Calories: 251g| Fat: 16g| Fiber: 3g| Carbs: 6g| Protein: 11 g

# Coriander Sausages Muffins

**Prep time: 10 minutes |Cook time: 12 minutes |Serves 4**

- 4 teaspoons coconut flour
- 1 tablespoon coconut cream
- 1 egg, beaten
- ½ teaspoon baking powder
- 6 oz sausage meat
- 1 teaspoon spring onions, chopped
- ½ teaspoon ground coriander
- 1 teaspoon sesame oil
- ½ teaspoon salt

1. In the mixing bowl mix up coconut flour, coconut cream, egg, baking powder, minced onion, and ground coriander.
2. Place the rack in the air fryer basket. Put the muffins on a rack.
3. Cook the meal for 12 minutes.

**PER SERVING**

Calories: 239g| Fat: 17.2g| Fiber: 5.1g| Carbs: 8.7g| Protein: 11.7g

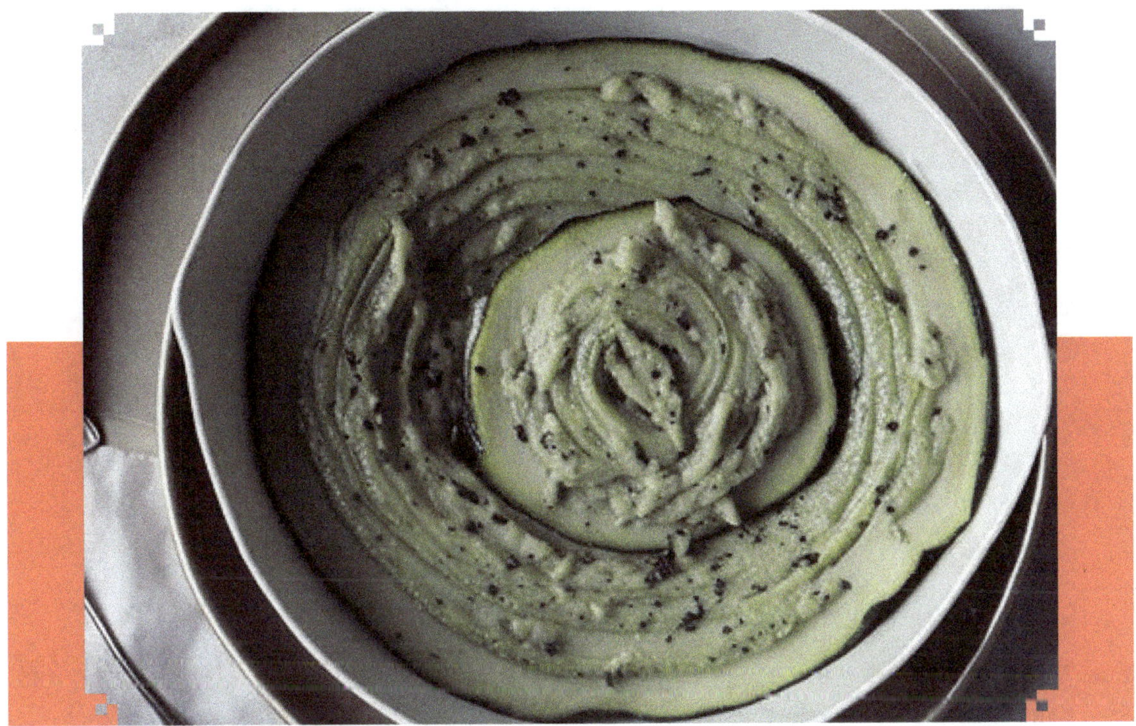

# Cheddar Tomatoes Hash

**Prep time: 5 minutes |Cook time: 25 minutes |Serves 4**

- 2 tablespoons olive oil
- 1 pound tomatoes, chopped
- ½ pound cheddar, shredded
- salt and black pepper to the taste
- 6 eggs, whisked

1. Add the oil to your air fryer, heat it up at 350 °F, add the tomatoes, eggs, salt and pepper and whisk.
2. Cook for 25 minutes, divide between plates and serve for breakfast.

**PER SERVING**

Calories: 221g| Fat: 8g| Fiber: 3g| Carbs: 4g| Protein: 8g

# Garlic Zucchini Spread

**Prep time: 10 minutes | Cook time: 15 minutes | Serves 4**

- 4 zucchinis, roughly chopped
- 1 teaspoon garlic powder
- 1 tablespoon avocado oil
- ½ teaspoon salt

1. Mix zucchini with garlic powder, avocado oil, and salt.
2. Put the mixture in the air fryer and bake at 375°F for 15 minutes.
3. Then blend the cooked zucchini until you get smooth spread.

**PER SERVING**

Calories: 38 | Fat: 0.8g | Fiber: 2.4g | Carbs: 7.3g | Protein: 2.5 g

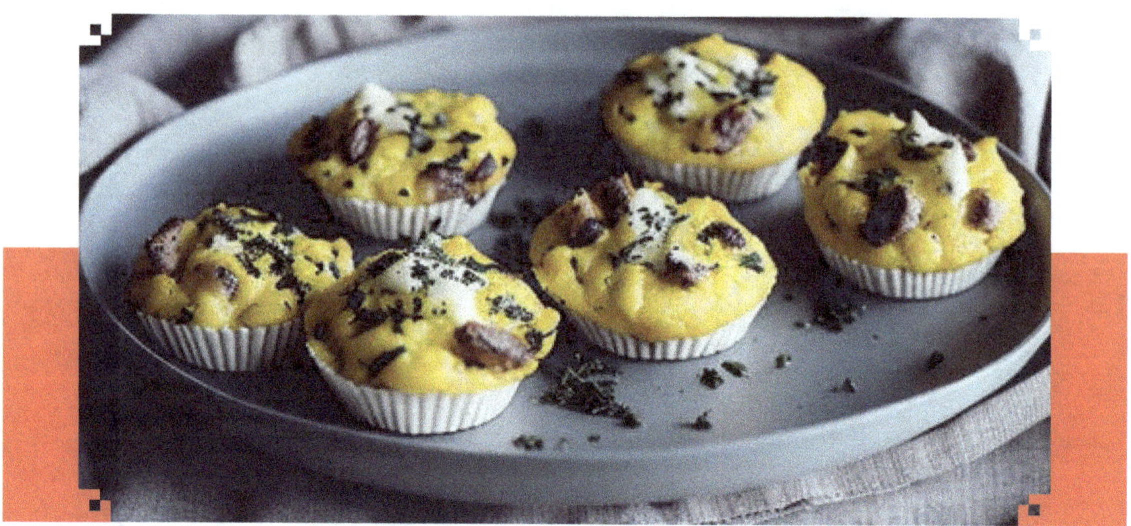

## Butter Donuts

**Prep time: 20 minutes |Cook time: 10 minutes |Serves 4**

- 1 cup almond flour
- 1 tablespoon flax meal
- 2 tablespoons erythritol
- 1 teaspoon baking powder
- 1 tablespoon psyllium husk powder

1. Make the dough: mix up almond flour, flax meal, eggs, baking powder, vanilla extract, heavy cream, and butter.
2. Add Psyllium husk and knead the soft but non-sticky dough. Then make the donuts balls and leave them for 10 minutes in a warm place.
3. Preheat the air fryer to 355F. Line the air fryer basket with baking paper.
4. Put the donuts inside and cook them brown. Then coat every donut in Erythritol.

**PER SERVING**

Calories: 103g| Fat: 7.8g| Fiber: 3g| Carbs: 4.9g| Protein: 4.7 g

## Scrambled Egg Muffins with Cheese

**Prep time: 10 minutes | Cook time: 20 minutes | Serves 6**

- 6 ounces smoked turkey sausage, chopped
- 6 eggs, lightly beaten
- 2 tablespoons shallots, finely chopped
- 2 garlic cloves, minced
- 1 teaspoon cayenne pepper
- 6 ounces Monterey Jack cheese, shredded

1. Simply combine the sausage, eggs, shallots, garlic, salt, black pepper, and cayenne pepper in a mixing dish. Mix to combine well.
2. Spoon the mixture into 6 standard-size muffin cups with paper liners.
3. Bake in the preheated Air Fryer at 340 °F for 8 minutes. Top with the cheese and bake an additional 8 minutes. Enjoy!

**PER SERVING**

Calories: 234 | Fat: 15.7g | Carbs: 5.3g | Protein: 17.6g | Fiber: 0.4g

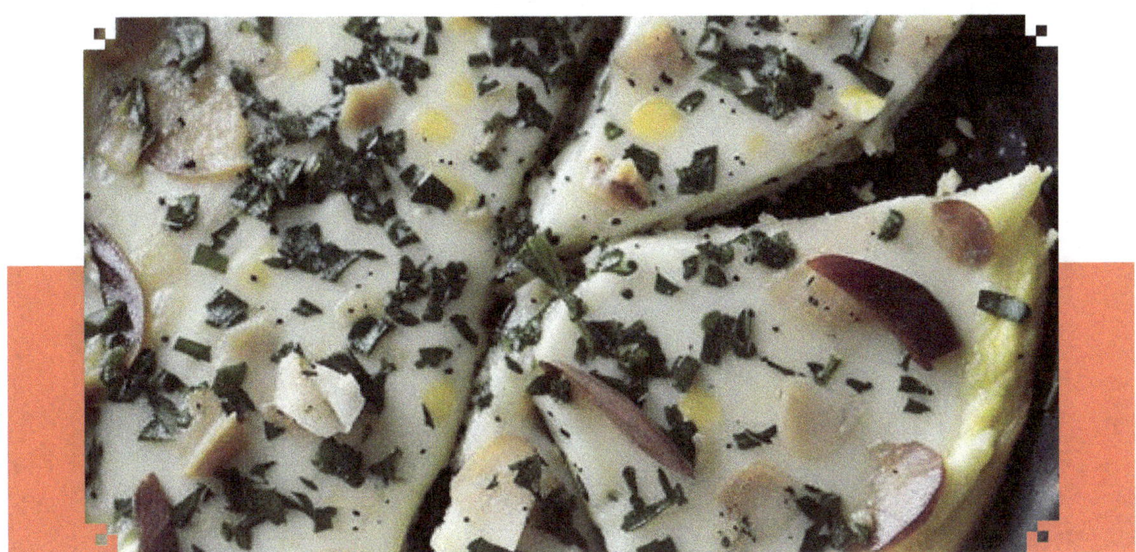

## Southwestern Breakfast Taco

**Prep time: 10 minutes | Cook time: 9 minutes |**
**Serves 1**

- 1 large egg, beaten
- ½ cup shredded mozzarella cheese
- 2 strips cooked bacon, crumbled
- ¼ avocado, diced
- hot sauce, for serving (optional)

1. In a medium bowl, whisk together the egg, mozzarella cheese, almond flour, chiles, taco seasoning, and baking powder.
2. Remove from the pan and top with the bacon, avocado, Cheddar cheese, sour cream, and salsa.
3. Serve warm with cilantro and hot sauce (if using).

**PER SERVING**

Calories: 563 | Fat: 42g | Carbs: 11g | Fiber: 5g | Protein: 34g

## Cod and Shallot Frittata

**Prep time: 10 minutes | Cook time: 20 minutes |**
**Serves 3**

- 2 cod fillets
- 6 eggs
- 1/2 cup milk
- 1 shallot, chopped
- 2 garlic cloves, minced
- 1/2 teaspoon red pepper flakes, crushed

1. Bring a pot of salted water to a boil. Boil the cod fillets for 5 minutes or until it is opaque. Flake the fish into bite-sized pieces.
2. Pour the mixture into the lightly greased baking pan.
3. Cook in the preheated Air Fryer at 360 °F for 9 minutes, flipping over halfway through. Bon appétit!

**PER SERVING**

Calories: 216 | Fat: 10g | Carbs: 5.2g | Protein: 24.4g | Fiber: 0.4g

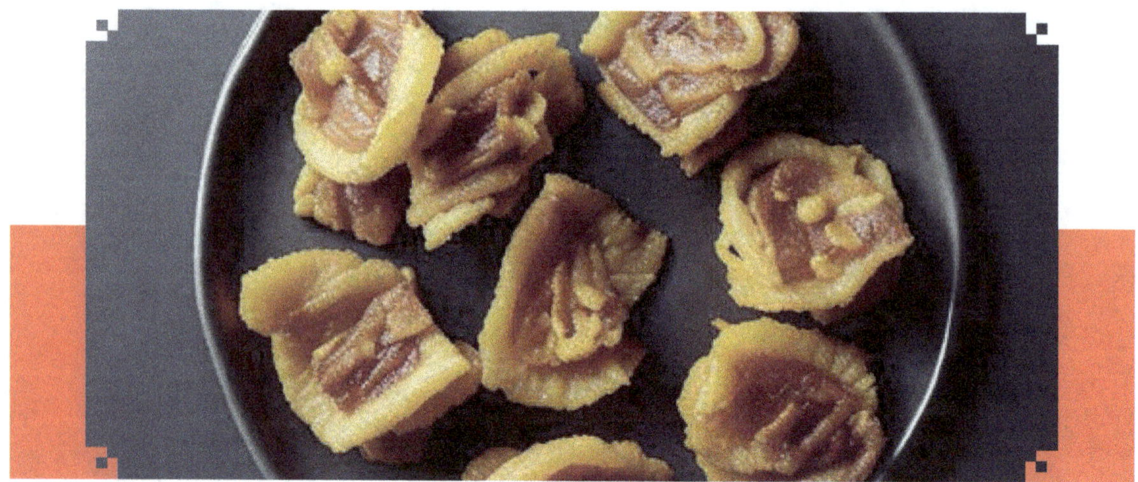

## Kale Omelet

**Prep time: 10 minutes |Cook time: 20 minutes |Serves 4**

- 1 eggplant, cubed
- 4 eggs, whisked
- 2 teaspoons cilantro, chopped
- salt and black pepper to the taste
- cooking spray
- ½ cup kale, chopped
- 2 tablespoons cheddar, grated
- 2 tablespoons fresh basil, chopped

1. In a bowl, mix all the ingredients except the cooking spray and whisk well.
2. Grease a pan that fits your air fryer with the cooking spray, pour the eggs mix, spread, put the pan in the machine and cook at 370 degrees F for 20 minutes.
3. Divide the mix between plates and serve for breakfast.

**PER SERVING**

Calories: 241g| Fat: 11g| Fiber: 4g| Carbs: 5g| Protein: 12g

## Fried Bacon

**Prep time: 10 minutes |Cook time: 12 minutes |Serves 4**

- 10 oz bacon
- 3 oz pork rinds
- ½ teaspoon salt
- ½ teaspoon ground black pepper
- cooking spray

1. Cut the bacon into 4 cubes and sprinkle with salt and ground black pepper.
2. After this dip the bacon cubes in the beaten eggs and coat in the pork rinds.
3. Preheat the air fryer to 395F.Spray the air fryer basket with cooking spray and put the bacon cubes inside. Cook them for 6 minutes.
4. Then flip the bacon on another side and cook for 6 minutes more or until it is light brown.

**PER SERVING**

Calories: 537g| Fat: 39.4g| Fiber: 0.1g| Carbs: 1.4g| Protein: 42.7g

# Chapter 5

## Poultry

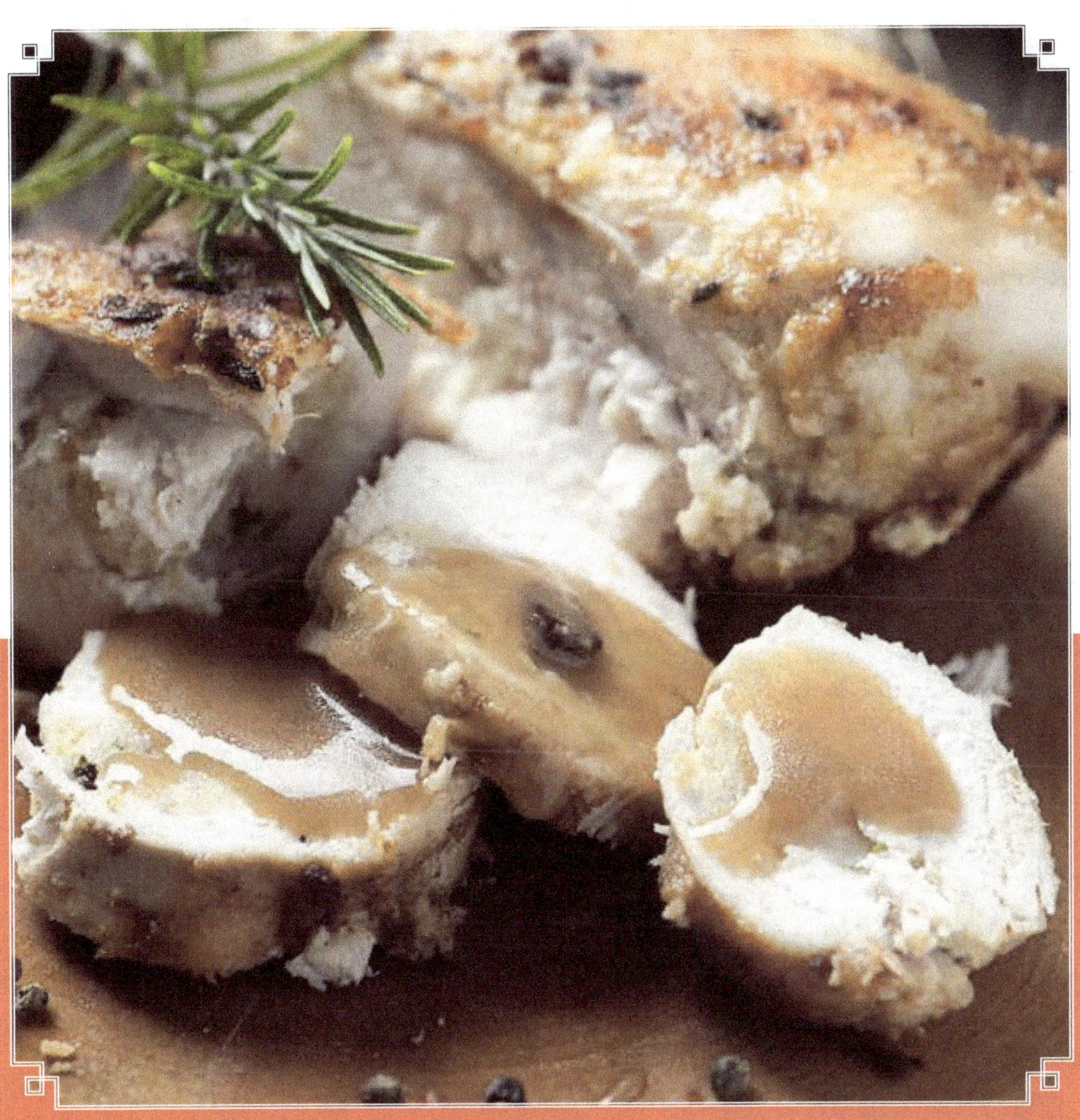

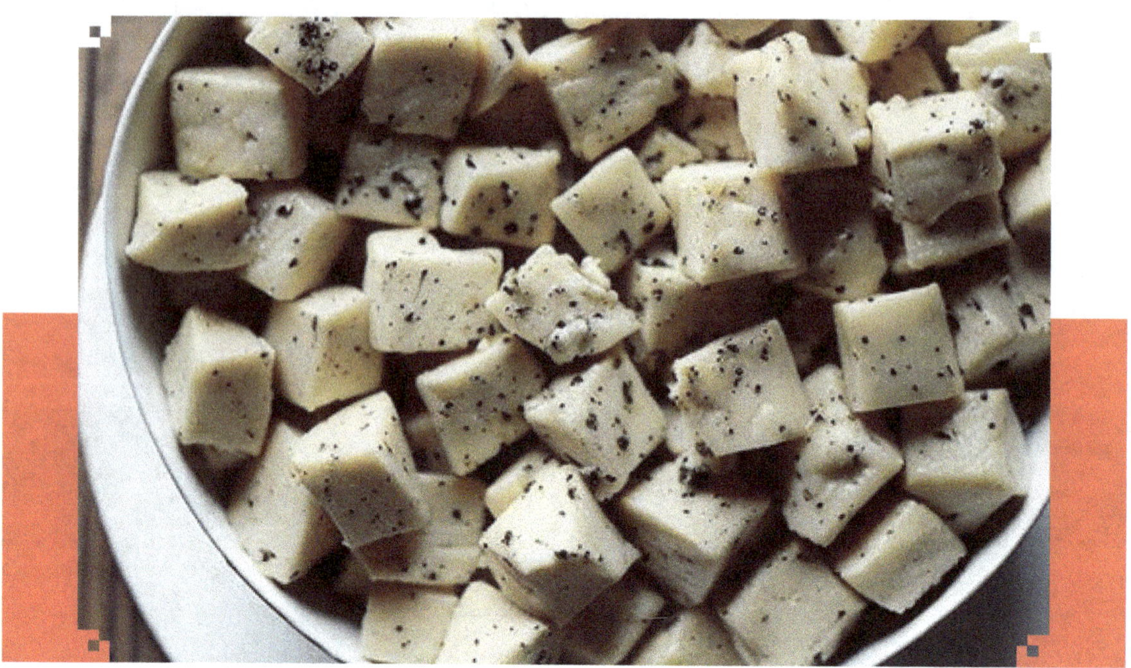

## Cilantro Turkey Casserole

**Prep time: 5 minutes |Cook time: 25 minutes |Serves 4**

- 2 tablespoons butter, melted
- 12 ounces cream cheese, soft
- 1 cups zucchinis, sliced
- 2 teaspoons sweet paprika
- ¼ cup cilantro, chopped
- salt and black pepper to the taste

1. In a baking dish that fits your air fryer, mix the butter with turkey, cream cheese and all the other ingredients except the cheddar cheese.
2. Divide between plates and serve for lunch.

**PER SERVING**

Calories: 280g| Fat: 10g| Fiber: 2g| Carbs: 4g| Protein: 12 g

## Mustard Chicken Cubes

**Prep time: 5 minutes | Cook time: 20 minutes | Serves 4**

- 16 oz chicken breast, skinless, boneless, cubed
- 1 tablespoon avocado oil
- 1 teaspoon mustard
- 1 teaspoon cream cheese

1. In the mixing bowl, mix avocado oil with mustard and cream cheese.
2. When the mixture is smooth, add chicken cubes and mix well.
3. Transfer the chicken cubes in the air fryer basket and cook at 360°F for 20 minutes.

**PER SERVING**

Calories: 141 | Fat: 3.8g | Fiber: 0.3g | Carbs: 0.5g | Protein: 24.4 g

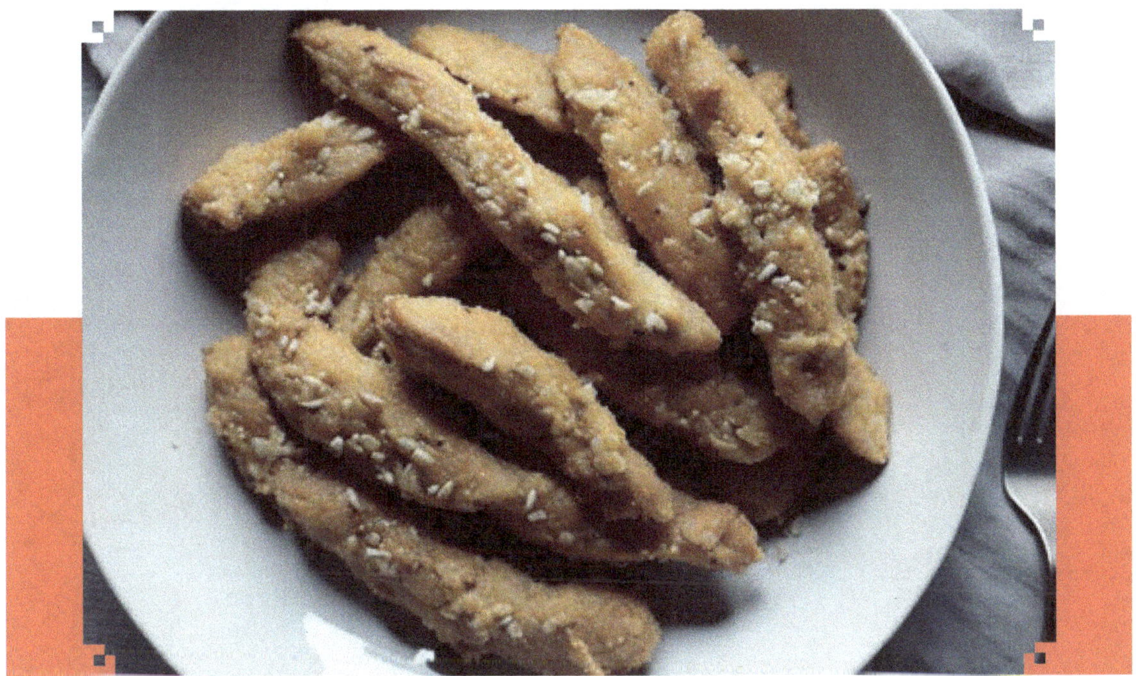

## Cayenne Pepper Chicken Halves

**Prep time: 10 minutes | Cook time: 30 minutes | Serves 4**

- 2-pounds chicken, halved
- 1 tablespoon cayenne pepper
- 1 tablespoon apple cider vinegar
- 1 tablespoon avocado oil

1. Rub the chicken halves with cayenne pepper, apple cider vinegar, and avocado oil.
2. Put the chicken halves in the air fryer and cook them at 360°F for 30 minutes per side.

**PER SERVING**

Calories: 352 | Fat: 7.5g | Fiber: 0.5g | Carbs: 1g | Protein: 65.9 g

## Almond Coconut Chicken Tenders

**Prep time: 5 minutes |Cook time: 20 minutes |Serves 4**

- a pinch of salt and black pepper
- 1/3 cup almond flour
- 2 eggs, whisked
- 9 ounces coconut flakes

1. Season the chicken tenders with salt and pepper, dredge them in almond flour, then dip in eggs and roll in coconut flakes.
2. Divide between plates and serve with a side salad.

**PER SERVING**

Calories: 250g| Fat: 12g| Fiber: 4g| Carbs: 6g| Protein: 15 g

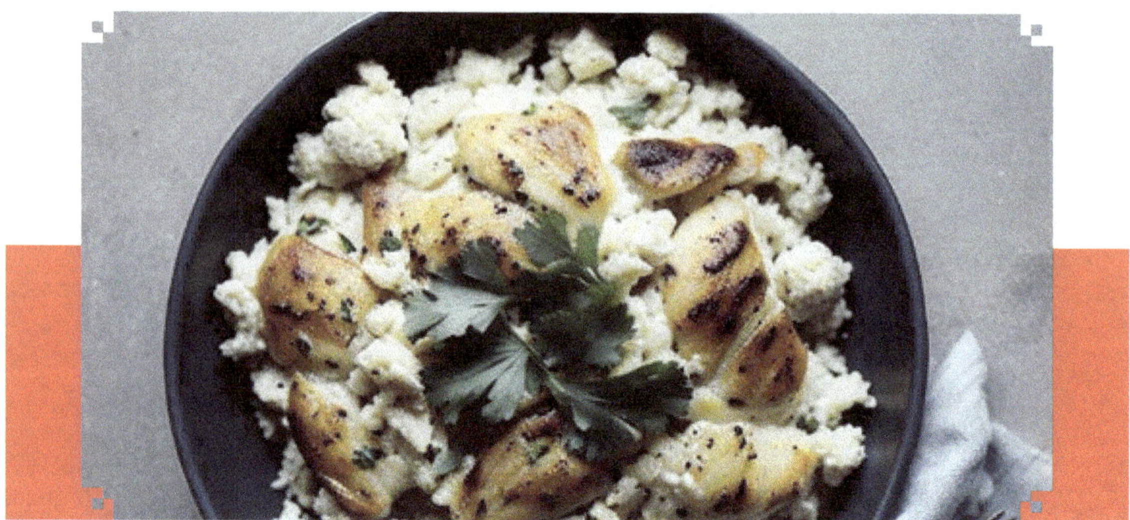

## Turkey and Lime Gravy

**Prep time: 5 minutes |Cook time: 25 minutes |Serves 4**

- 1 big turkey breast, skinless, boneless, cubed and browned
- juice of 1 lime
- zest of 1 lime, grated
- 1 cup chicken stock
- 2 tablespoons thyme, chopped
- a pinch of salt and black pepper

1. Heat up a pan that fits the air fryer with the butter over medium heat, add all the ingredients except the turkey, whisk, bring to a simmer and cook for 5 minutes.
2. Add the turkey cubes, put the pan in the air fryer and cook at 380 °F for 20 minutes.
3. Divide the meat between plates, drizzle the gravy all over and serve.

**PER SERVING**

Calories: 284g| Fat: 13g| Fiber: 3g| Carbs: 5g| Protein: 15 g

## Chicken and Rice Casserole

**Prep time: 5 minutes |Cook time: 35 minutes |Serves 4**

- 2 cups cauliflower florets, chopped
- a pinch of salt and black pepper
- a drizzle of olive oil
- 6 ounces coconut cream
- 2 teaspoons thyme, chopped
- 1 tablespoon parsley, chopped
- 4 chicken thighs, boneless and skinless

1. Heat up a pan with the butter over medium heat, add the cream and the other ingredients except the cauliflower, oil and the chicken, whisk, bring to a simmer and cook for 5 minutes.
2. Heat up a pan with the oil over medium-high heat, add the chicken and brown for 2 minutes on each side.
3. Divide between plates and serve hot.

**PER SERVING**

Calories: 280g| Fat: 14g| Fiber: 4g| Carbs: 6g| Protein: 20g

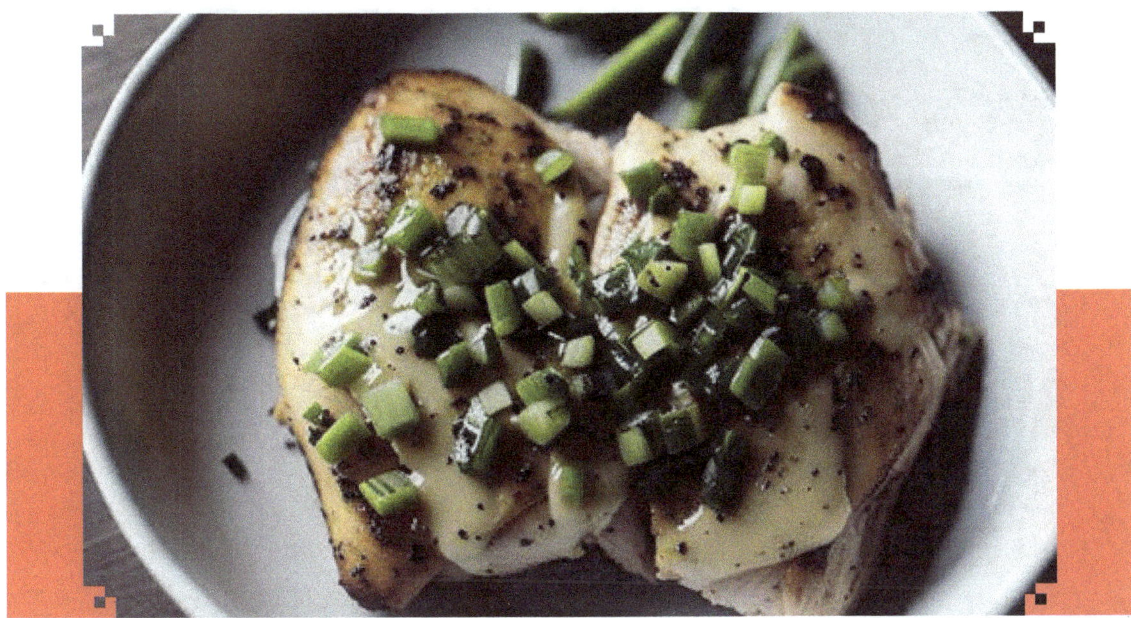

## Jalapeño Popper Chicken

**Prep time: 10 minutes | Cook time: 14 to 17 minutes | Serves 8**

- 2 pounds boneless, skinless chicken breasts or thighs
- 4 ounces cheddar cheese, shredded
- 1 teaspoon minced garlic
- avocado oil spray

1. Place the chicken in a large zip-top bag or between two pieces of plastic wrap. Season both sides of the chicken with salt and pepper.
2. Set the air fryer to 350°F. Spray the outside of the chicken with oil. Flip to 10 minutes, until an instant-read thermometer reads 160°F.

**PER SERVING**

Calories: 264 | Fat: 17g |Carbs: 2g | Fiber: 1g | Protein: 28g

## Cream Cheese Chicken

**Prep time: 10 minutes | Cook time: 25 minutes | Serves 5**

- 1½-pound chicken breast, skinless, boneless
- 1 teaspoon ground paprika
- ½ teaspoon ground turmeric
- 2 teaspoons cream cheese
- 1 oz scallions, chopped
- 1 teaspoon avocado oil
- ½ teaspoon salt

1. Rub the chicken breast with ground paprika, turmeric, and salt.
2. Then put the chicken in the air fryer basket.
3. Add avocado oil, scallions, and cream cheese.
4. Cook the meal at 375°F for 25 minutes.

**PER SERVING**

Calories: 165 | Fat: 4.1g | Fiber: 0.4g | Carbs: 0.9g | Protein: 29.1 g

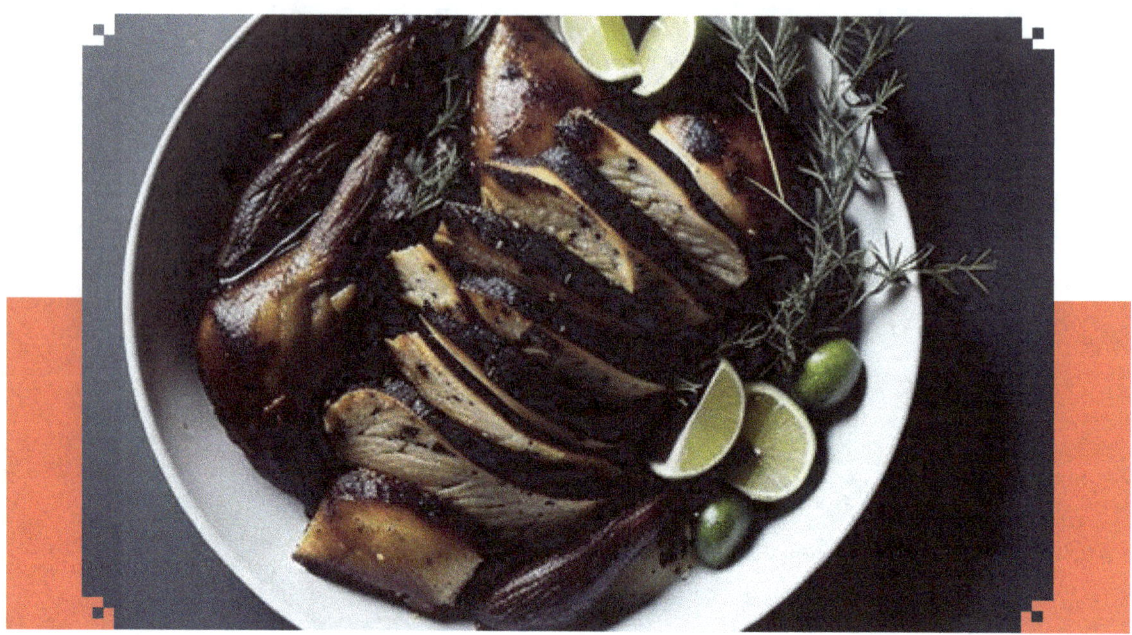

## Lemon-Dijon Boneless Chicken

**Prep time: 5 minutes, plus 30 minutes to 4 hours to marinate | Cook time: 13 to 16 minutes | Serves 6**

- 1 tablespoon dijon mustard
- 1 teaspoon sea salt
- ½ teaspoon freshly ground black pepper
- ¼ teaspoon cayenne pepper

1. In a small bowl, combine the mayonnaise, mustard, lemon juice seasoning, salt, black pepper, and cayenne pepper.
2. Set the air fryer to 400°F. Flip the 9 minutes more, until an instant-read thermometer reads 160°F.

**PER SERVING**

Calories: 236 |Fat: 17g | Carbs: 1g | Fiber: 1g |Protein: 23g

## Lime and Thyme Duck

**Prep time: 15 minutes |Cook time: 17 minutes |Serves 4**

- 1-pound duck breast, skinless, boneless
- 2 oz preserved lime, sliced
- 1 teaspoon apple cider vinegar
- 1 tablespoon olive oil
- ½ teaspoon dried thyme

1. Cut the duck breast on 4 pieces and sprinkle with salt, dried thyme, apple cider vinegar, and oil.
2. Mix up the duck pieces well and put on the foil the duck and wrap the foil.
3. Preheat the air fryer to 375°F and put fryer basket.
4. Cook it for 17 minutes.

**PER SERVING**

Calories: 184g| Fat: 8.4g| Fiber: 0.1g| Carbs: 1.1g| Protein: 25 g

# Chapter 6

## Beef, Pork and Lamb

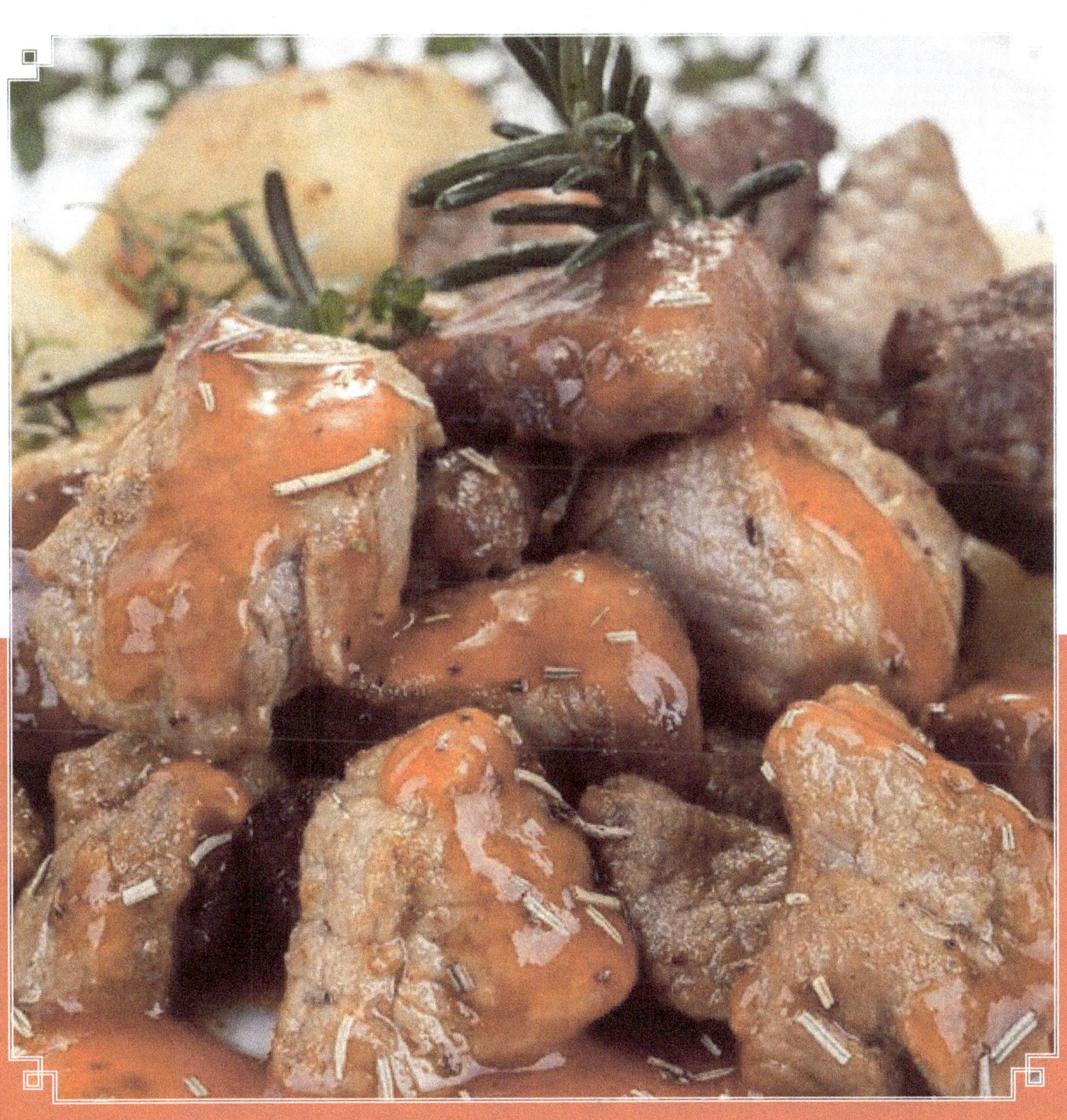

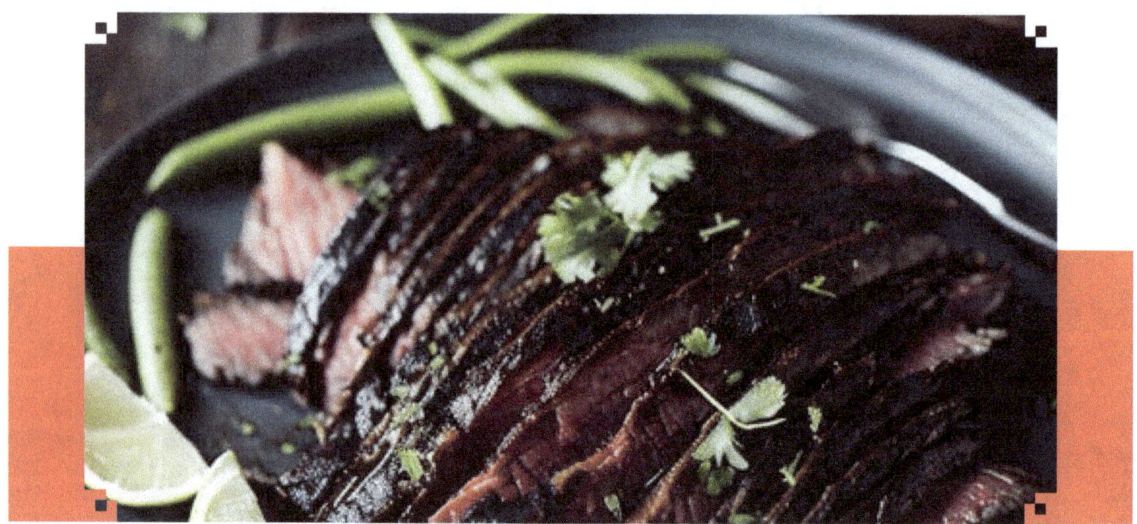

## Pork and Mushrooms Mix

**Prep time: 5 minutes |Cook time: 20 minutes |Serves 4**

- 1 pound pork stew meat, ground
- 1 cup mushrooms, sliced
- 2 spring onions, chopped
- salt and black pepper to the taste
- 1 teaspoon Italian seasoning
- ½ teaspoon garlic powder
- 1 tablespoon olive oil

1. Heat up a pan that fits the air fryer with the oil over medium high heat, add the meat and brown for 3-4 minutes.
2. Add the rest of the ingredients, stir, put the pan in the Air Fryer, cover and cook at 360 °F for 15 minutes.
3. Divide between plates and serve for lunch.

**PER SERVING**

Calories: 220g| Fat: 12g| Fiber: 2g| Carbs: 4g| Protein: 7g

## BBQ Skirt Steak

**Prep time: 10 minutes | Cook time: 20 minutes | Serves 5**

- 2 pounds skirt steak
- 2 tablespoons tomato paste
- 1 tablespoon olive oil
- 1 tablespoon coconut aminos
- 1/4 cup rice vinegar
- 1 tablespoon fish sauce

1. Place all ingredients in a large ceramic dish; let it marinate for 3 hours in your refrigerator.
2. Coat the sides and bottom of the Air Fryer with cooking spray.
3. Add your steak to the cooking basket; reserve the marinade. Cook the skirt steak in the preheated Air Fryer at 400 °F for 12 basting with the reserved marinade.
4. Bon appétit!

**PER SERVING**

Calories: 401 | Fat: 21g | Carbs: 1.7g | Protein: 51g | Fiber: 1g

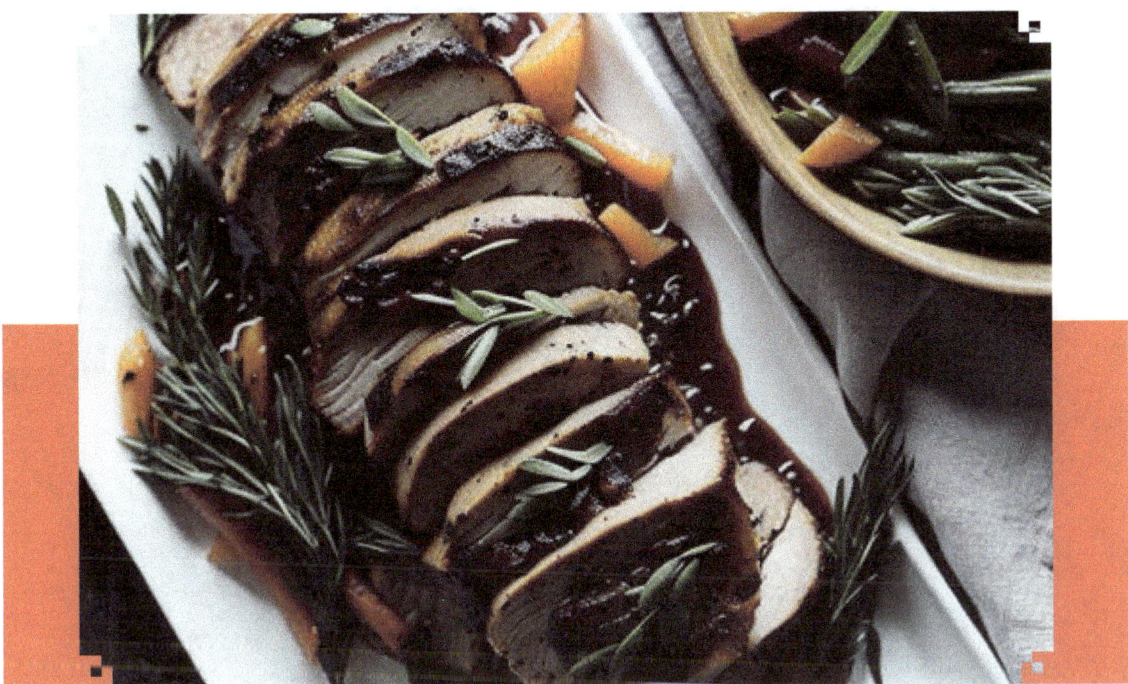

## Roasted Cilantro Lamb Chops

**Prep time: 5 minutes |Cook time: 24 minutes |Serves 6**

- 12 lamb chops
- a pinch of salt and black pepper
- juice of 1 lime
- 3 tablespoons olive oil

1. In a bowl, mix the lamb chops with the rest of the ingredients and rub well.
2. Put the chops in your air fryer's basket and cook at 400 °F for 12 minutes on each side. Divide between plates and serve.

**PER SERVING**

Calories: 284g| Fat: 10g| Fiber: 3g| Carbs: 6g| Protein: 16g

## Italian-Style Pork Loin Roast

**Prep time: 10 minutes | Cook time: 50 minutes | Serves 3**

- 1 teaspoon Celtic sea salt
- 1/4 cup red wine
- 1 pound pork top loin
- 1 tablespoon Italian herb seasoning blend

1. In a ceramic bowl, mix the salt, black pepper, red wine, mustard, and garlic. Add the pork top loin and let it marinate at least 30 minutes.
2. Cook the pork tenderloin at 370 °F for 10 minutes. Serve immediately.

**PER SERVING**

Calories: 300 | Fat: 9g | Carbs: 1.5g | Protein: 33.8g | Fiber: 0.5g

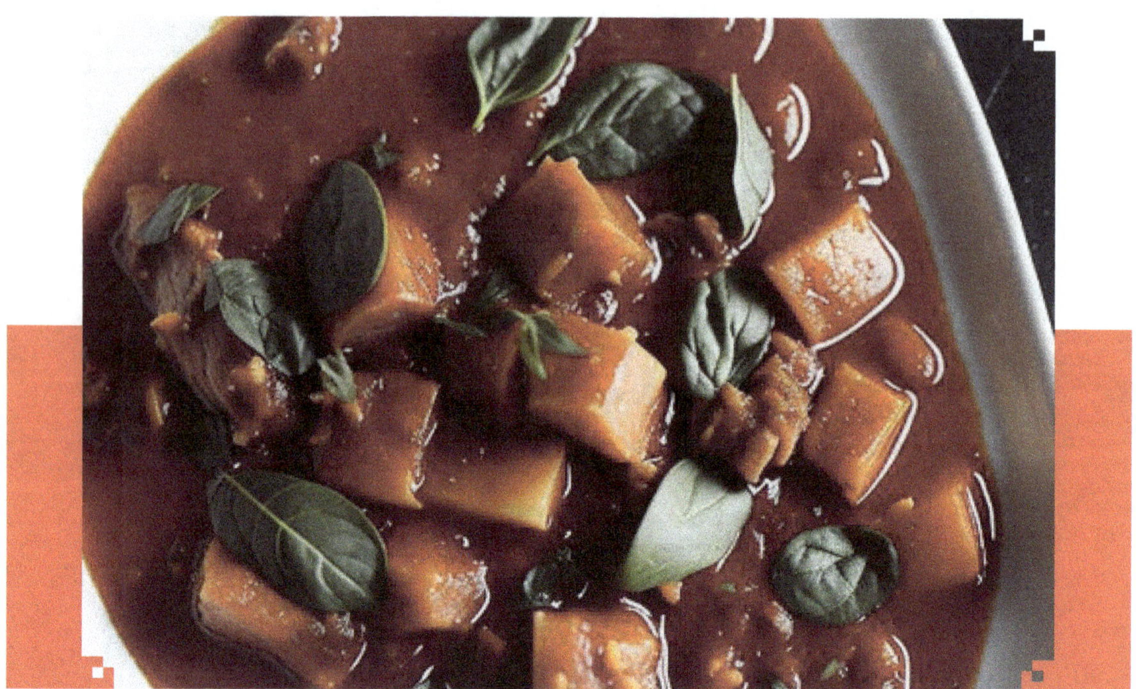

## Caraway Seeds Lamb Loin

**Prep time: 10 minutes | Cook time: 30 minutes | Serves 4**

- 2-pound lamb loin
- ½ cup apple cider vinegar
- 1 tablespoon coconut oil, melted
- 1 tablespoon caraway seeds
- ½ teaspoon salt

1. Marinate the lamb loin in the mixture of apple cider vinegar, coconut oil, caraway seeds, and salt.
2. Then put the meat in the air fryer and cook it at 375°F for 30 minutes.

### PER SERVING

Calories: 474 | Fat: 22.8g | Fiber: 0.8g | Carbs: 1.3g | Protein: 60.7 g

## Pork and Spinach Stew

**Prep time: 5 minutes |Cook time: 25 minutes |Serves 4**

- 1 pound pork stew meat, cubed
- 2 carrots, cubed
- 3 garlic cloves, minced
- ½ teaspoon olive oil

1. In pan that fits your air fryer, mix the pork with the other ingredients except the spinach, toss, introduce in the fryer and cook at 370 °F for 15 minutes.
2. Add the spinach, toss, cook for 10 minutes more, divide into bowls and serve for lunch.

### PER SERVING

Calories: 290g| Fat: 14g| Fiber: 3g| Carbs: 5g| Protein: 13 g

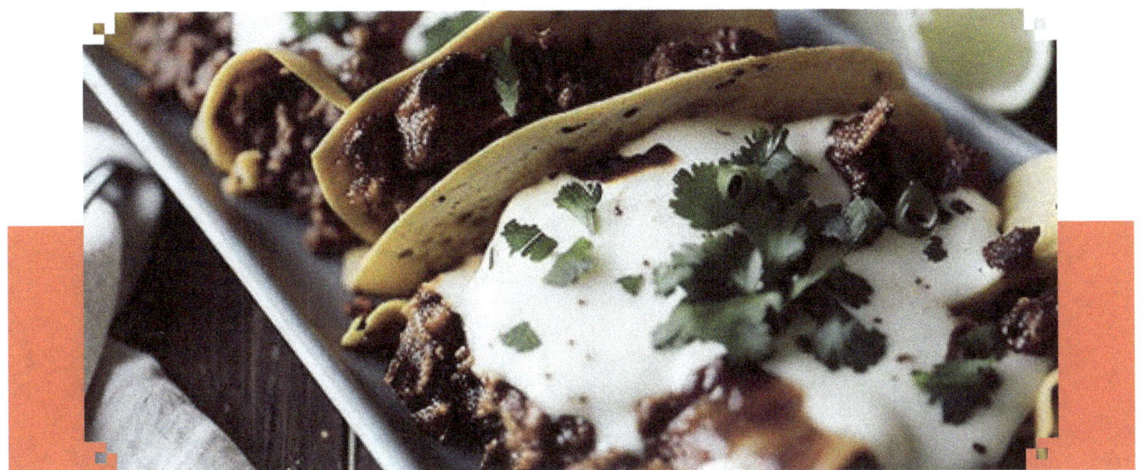

# Sweet and Spicy Spare Ribs

**Prep time: 10 minutes | Cook time: 30 minutes |**
**Serves 6**

- ¼ cup granular brown erythritol
- 2 teaspoons paprika
- 2 teaspoons chili powder
- 1 teaspoon garlic powder
- ½ teaspoon cayenne pepper
- 1 (4-pound) rack pork spare ribs

1. In a small bowl, mix erythritol, paprika, chili powder, garlic powder, cayenne pepper, salt, and black pepper. Rub spice mix over ribs on both sides. Place ribs on ungreased aluminum foil sheet and wrap to cover.
2. Place ribs into ungreased air fryer basket. Adjust the temperature to 400°F and set the timer for 25 minutes.
3. When timer beeps, remove ribs from foil, Serve warm.

## PER SERVING

Calories: 474 | Protein: 35g | Fiber: 1g | Carbs: 0g | Fat: 32g

# Beef and Green Onions Casserole

**Prep time: 15 minutes |Cook time: 21 minutes**
**|Serves 4**

- 10 oz lean ground beef
- 1 oz green onions, chopped
- 2 low carb tortillas
- 1 tablespoon mascarpone
- 1 tablespoon heavy cream
- 1 teaspoon olive oil

1. Pour olive oil in the skillet and heat it up over the medium heat. Then add ground beef and sprinkle it with garlic powder and Mexican seasonings.
2. Secure the edges of the pan well. Preheat the air fryer to 360°F.
3. Cook the casserole for 10 minutes at 360°F and then remove the baking paper and cook the meal for 5 minutes more to reach the crunchy crust.

## PER SERVING

Calories: 179g| Fat: 14.7g| Fiber: 3g| Carbs: 6.6g| Protein: 23.8 g

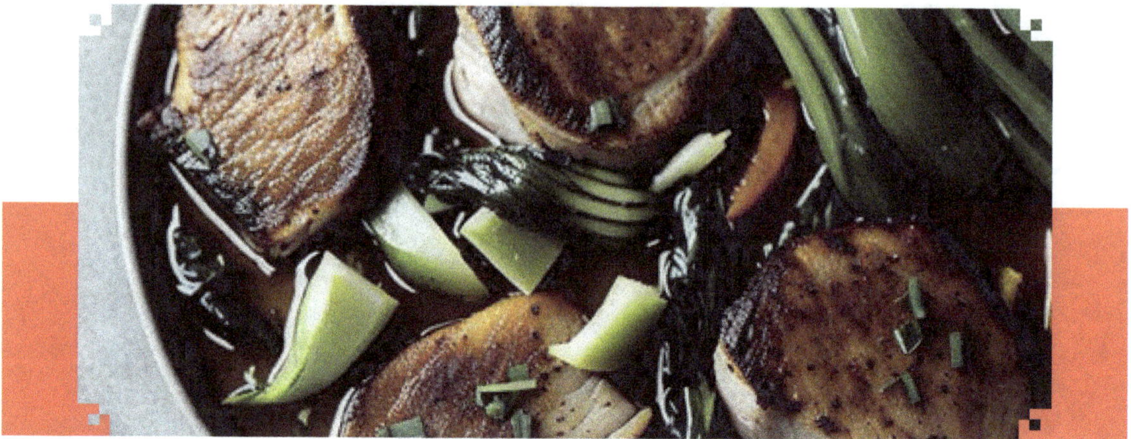

## Goat Cheese-Stuffed Flank Steak

**Prep time: 10 minutes | Cook time: 14 minutes | Serves 6**

- 1 pound flank steak
- 1 tablespoon avocado oil
- ½ teaspoon sea salt
- ½ teaspoon garlic powder
- 1 cup baby spinach, chopped

1. Place the steak in a large zip-top bag or between two pieces of plastic wrap. Using a meat mallet or heavy-bottomed skillet, pound the steak to an even ¼-inch thickness.
2. Brush both sides of the steak with the avocado oil.
3. Set the air fryer to 400°F. Flip the steak and cook for an additional 7 minutes, until an instant-read thermometer reads 120°F for medium-rare (adjust the cooking time for your desired doneness).

**PER SERVING**

Calories: 165 | Fat: 9g | Carbs: 1g | Fiber: 1g | Protein: 18g

## Garlic Pork and Bok Choy

**Prep time: 5 minutes |Cook time: 35 minutes |Serves 4**

- 4 pork chops, boneless
- 1 bok choy head, torn
- 2 cups chicken stock
- 2 tablespoons coconut aminos
- 2 garlic cloves, minced
- 2 tablespoons coconut oil, melted

1. Heat up a pan that fits the air fryer with the oil over medium-high heat, add the pork chops and brown for 5 minutes.
2. Add the garlic, salt and pepper and cook for another minute. Add the rest of the ingredients except the bok choy and cook at 380 degrees F for 25 minutes.
3. Add the bok choy, cook for 5 minutes more, divide everything between plates and serve.

**PER SERVING**

Calories: 284g| Fat: 14g| Fiber: 4g| Carbs: 6g| Protein: 17g

# Chapter 7

## Fish & Seafood

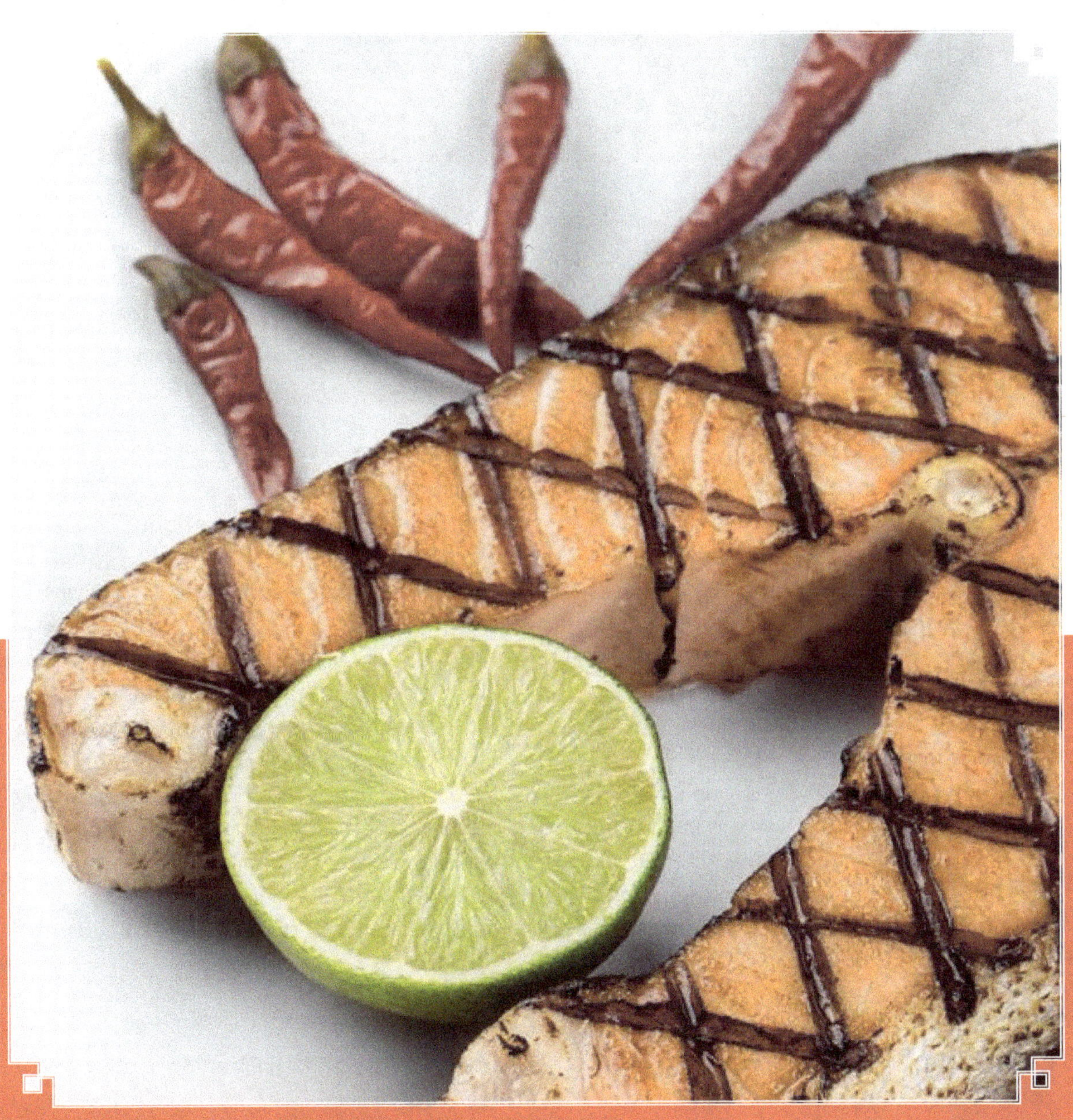

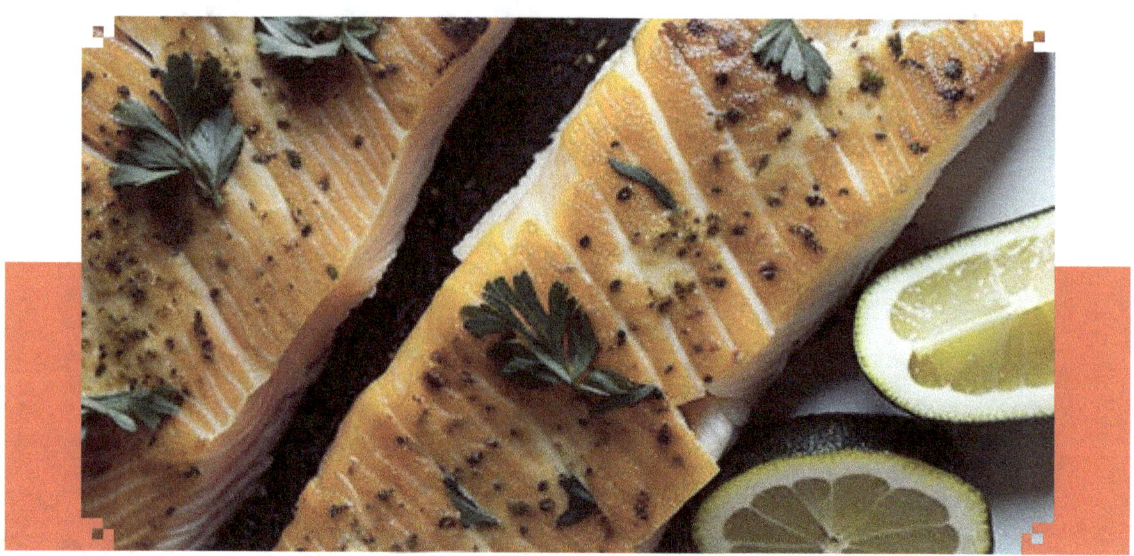

# Shrimp and Mushroom Pie

**Prep time: 15 minutes |Cook time: 15 minutes |Serves 4**

- 10 oz shrimps, peeled
- ½ cup cheddar cheese, shredded
- 3 tablespoons cream cheese
- 2 eggs, beaten
- ¼ cup cremini mushrooms, sliced
- ½ teaspoon salt
- 1 teaspoon nut oil

1. Mix up shrimps and seafood seasonings.
2. Then brush the air fryer round pan with nut oil and put the shrimps inside.
3. Pour the mixture over the shrimps and flatten the pie gently with the help of the fork or spoon. Cook the shrimp pie for 15 minutes.

**PER SERVING**

Calories: 211g| Fat: 11.8g| Fiber: 0.1g| Carbs: 2g| Protein: 23.1 gg

# Parmesan Salmon Fillets

**Prep time: 5 minutes |Cook time: 15 minutes |Serves 4**

- 4 salmon fillets, skinless
- 1 teaspoon mustard
- a pinch of salt and black pepper
- ½ cup coconut flakes
- 1 tablespoon parmesan, grated
- cooking spray

1. In a bowl, mix the parmesan with the other ingredients except the fish and cooking spray and stir well.
2. Coat the fish in this mix, grease it with cooking spray and arrange in the air fryer's basket.
3. Cook at 400 °F for 15 minutes, divide between plates and serve with a side salad.

**PER SERVING**

Calories: 240g| Fat: 13g| Fiber: 3g| Carbs: 6g| Protein: 15g

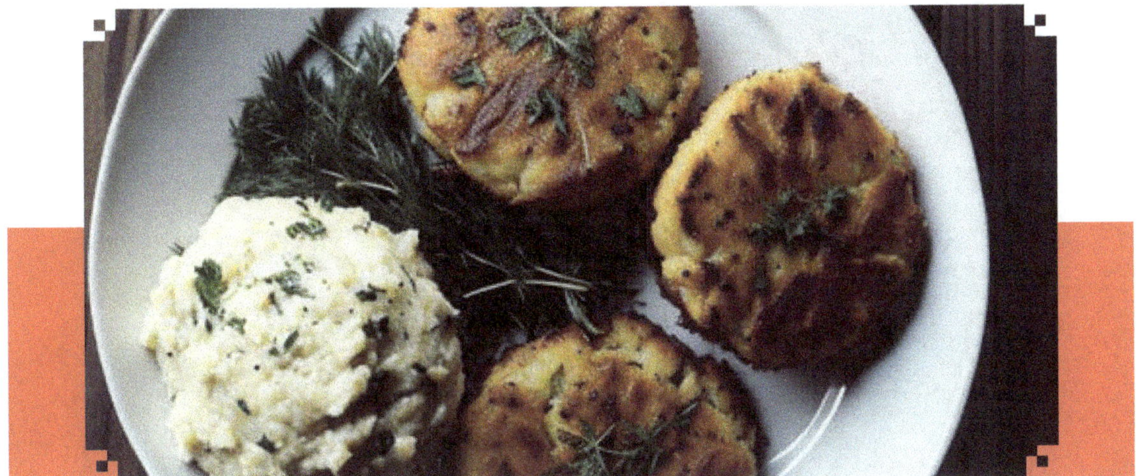

## Crispy Parmesan Lobster Tails

**Prep time: 5 minutes | Cook time: 7 minutes | Serves 4**

- 4 (4-ounce) lobster tails
- 2 tablespoons salted butter, melted
- ¼ teaspoon salt
- ¼ cup grated parmesan cheese
- ½ ounce plain pork rinds, finely crushed

1. Cut lobster tails open carefully with a pair of scissors and gently pull meat away from shells, resting meat on top of shells.
2. Brush lobster meat with butter and sprinkle with 1 teaspoon Cajun seasoning, ¼ teaspoon per tail.
3. Carefully place tails into ungreased air fryer basket. Lobster tails will be internal temperature of at least 145°F when done. Serve warm.

**PER SERVING**

Calories: 184 | Protein: 23g | Fiber: 0g | Carbs: 1g | Fat: 9g

## Dilled Crab and Cauliflower Cakes

**Prep time: 10 minutes | Cook time: 20 minutes | Serves 4**

- 1 ½ tablespoons mayonnaise
- 1/2 teaspoon whole-grain mustard
- 2 eggs, well beaten
- 1/3 teaspoon ground black pepper
- 1/2 pound cup mashed cauliflower
- 1/2 teaspoon dried dill weed
- 1/2 pound crabmeat
- A pinch of salt
- 1 ½ tablespoons softened butter

1. Mix all the ingredients thoroughly. Shape into 4 patties.
2. Then, spritz your patties with cooking oil.
3. Air-fry at 365 °F for 12 minutes, turning halfway through. Serve over boiled potatoes. Bon appétit!

**PER SERVING**

Calories: 184 | Fat: 11.6g | Carbs: 3.2g | Protein: 16.2g | Fiber: 1.4g

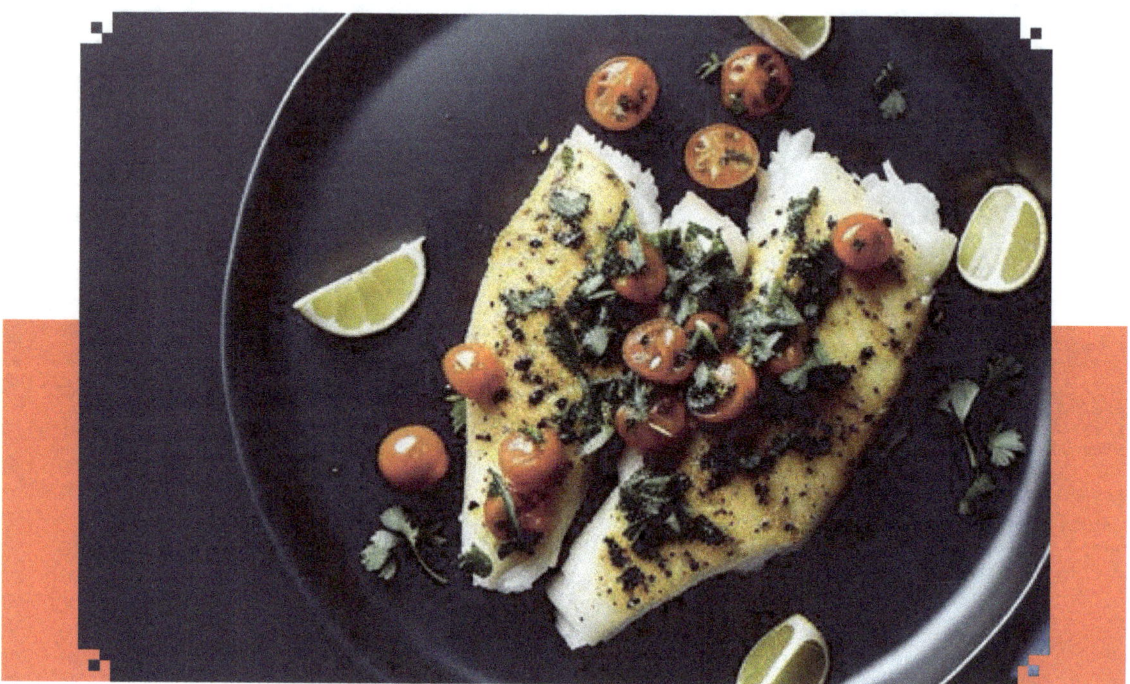

# Chipotle Salmon Fish Cakes

**Prep time: 10 minutes | Cook time: 2 hours 15 minutes | Serves 4**

- 1/2 teaspoon chipotle powder
- 1/2 teaspoon butter, at room temperature
- 2 tablespoons coconut flour
- 2 tablespoons parmesan cheese, grated

1. Place all ingredients in a large-sized mixing dish.
2. Shape into cakes and roll each cake over seasoned breadcrumbs. After that, refrigerate for about 2 hours.
3. Serve warm with a dollop of sour cream if desired. Bon appétit!

**PER SERVING**

Calories: 401 | Fat: 19.4g | Carbs: 2g | Protein: 53g | Fiber: 0.5g

# Cilantro Cod Mix

**Prep time: 5 minutes |Cook time: 15 minutes |Serves 4**

- 1 cup cherry tomatoes, halved
- salt and black pepper to the taste
- 2 tablespoons olive oil
- 4 cod fillets, skinless and boneless
- 2 tablespoons cilantro, chopped

1. In a baking dish that fits your air fryer, mix all the ingredients, toss gently, introduce in your air fryer and cook at 370 °F for 15 minutes.
2. Divide everything between plates and serve right away.

**PER SERVING**

Calories: 248g| Fat: 11g| Fiber: 2g| Carbs: 5g| Protein: 11g

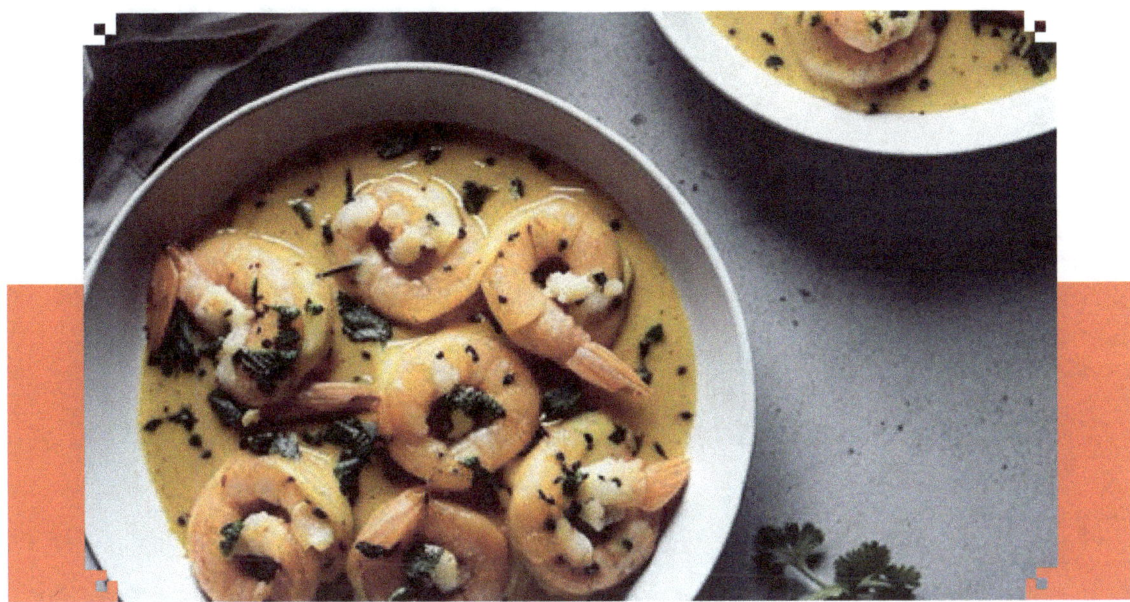

## Sesame-Crusted Salmon

**Prep time: 15 minutes | Cook time: 10 minutes |**
Serves 4

- 1 tablespoon reduced-sodium soy sauce
- 1 teaspoon sesame oil
- 1 teaspoon honey
- 2 tablespoons chopped fresh marjoram, for garnish (optional)

1. Preheat the air fryer to 360°F.
2. Place the sesame seeds on a plate or small bowl, combine the soy sauce, sesame oil, and honey.
3. Arrange the fish in a single layer in the basket of the air fryer, seed-side up. Top with the marjoram, if desired, before serving.

**PER SERVING**

Calories: 310 | Protein: 35g | Carbs: 3g| Fat: 17g | Fiber: 1g

## Cheesy Shrimp Bake

**Prep time: 15 minutes | Cook time: 5 minutes |**
Serves 4

- 14 oz shrimps, peeled
- 1 egg, beaten
- ½ cup of coconut milk
- 1 cup Cheddar cheese, shredded
- ½ teaspoon coconut oil
- 1 teaspoon ground coriander

1. In the mixing bowl, mix shrimps with egg, coconut milk, Cheddar cheese, coconut oil, and ground coriander.
2. Then put the mixture in the baking ramekins and put in the air fryer.
3. Cook the shrimps at 400°F for 5 minutes.

**PER SERVING**

Calories: 321 | Fat: 19.9g | Fiber: 0.7g | Carbs: 3.6g | Protein: 31.7 g

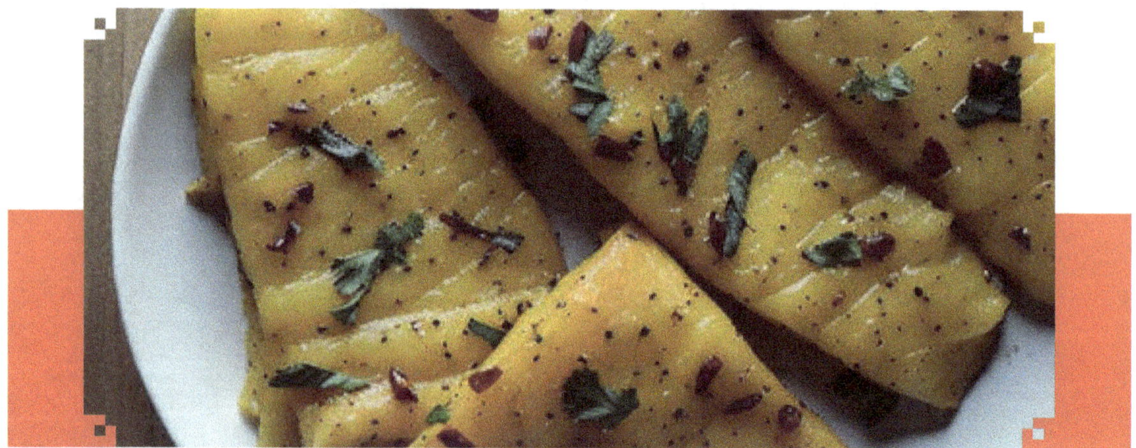

# Italian Eggs with Smoked Salmon

**Prep time: 10 minutes | Cook time: 25 minutes | Serves 4**

- 1/3 cup Asiago cheese, grated
- 1/3 teaspoon dried dill weed
- 1/2 tomato, chopped
- 6 eggs
- 1/3 cup milk
- Pan spray
- 1/3 teaspoon smoked cayenne pepper

1. Set your air fryer to cook at 365 °F. In a mixing bowl, whisk the eggs, milk, smoked cayenne pepper, salt, black pepper, and dill weed.
2. Lightly grease 4 ramekins with pan spray of choice; divide the egg/milk mixture among the prepared ramekins.
3. Add the salmon and tomato; top with the grated Asiago cheese. Finally, air-fry for 16 minutes. Bon appétit!

**PER SERVING**

Calories: 310 | Fat: 17.2g | Carbs: 2.1g | Protein: 33.2g | Fiber: 0.2g

# Fijan Coconut Fish

**Prep time: 10 minutes | Cook time: 20 minutes | Serves 2**

- 1 cup coconut milk
- 2 tablespoons lime juice
- 2 tablespoons Shoyu sauce
- Salt and white pepper, to taste
- 1 pound tilapia
- 2 tablespoons olive oil

1. In a mixing bowl, thoroughly combine the coconut milk with the lime juice, Shoyu sauce, salt, pepper, turmeric, ginger, and chili pepper. Add tilapia and let it marinate for 1 hour.
2. Brush the Air Fryer basket with olive oil. tilapia fillets in the Air Fryer basket.
3. Cook the tilapia in the preheated Air over and cook for 6 minutes more. Work in batches.
4. Serve with some extra lime wedges if desired. Enjoy!

**PER SERVING**

Calories: 426 | Fat: 21.5g | Carbs: 9.4g | Protein: 50.2g | Fiber: 3.4g

# Chapter 8

## Side Dishes and Snacks

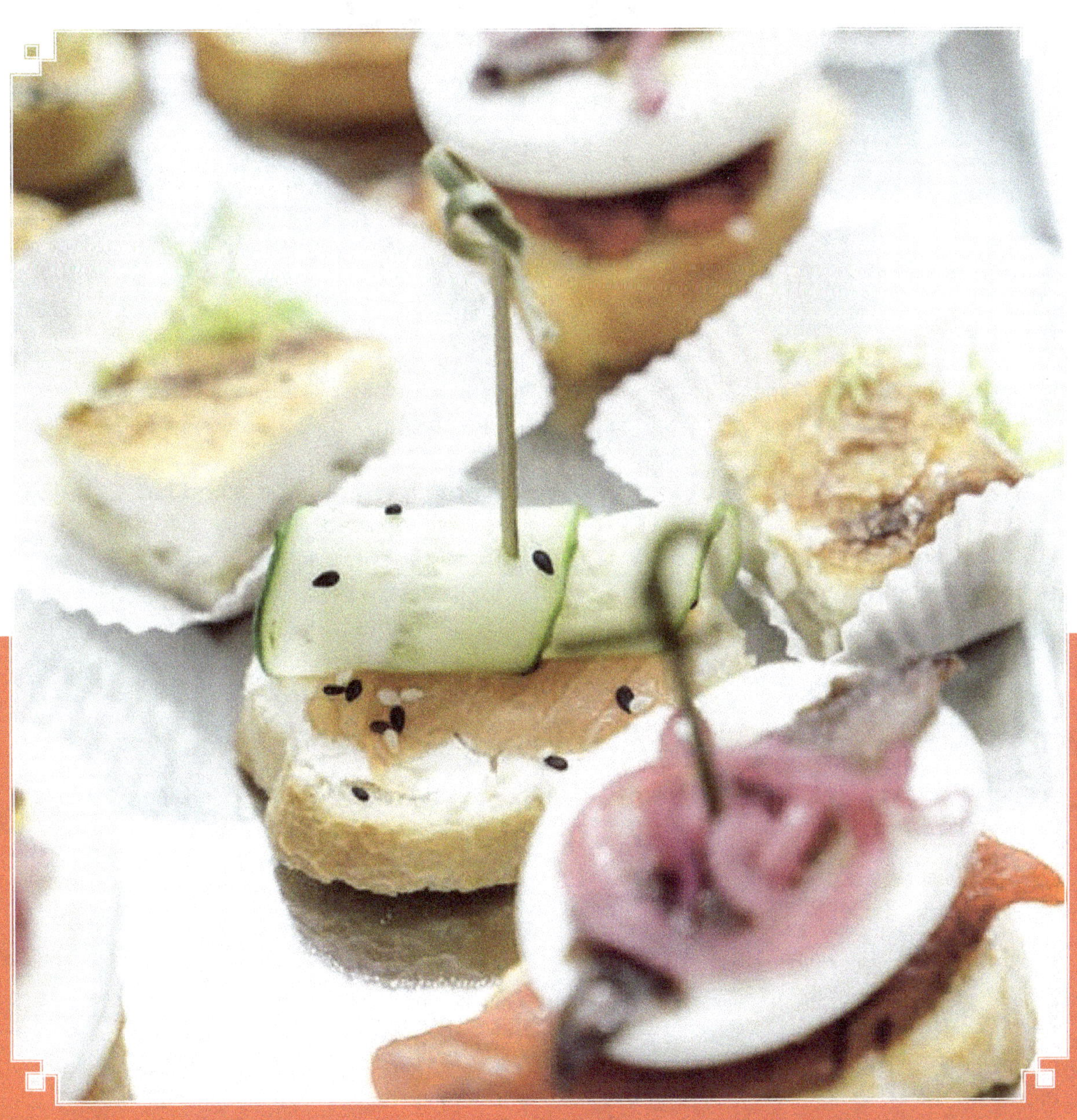

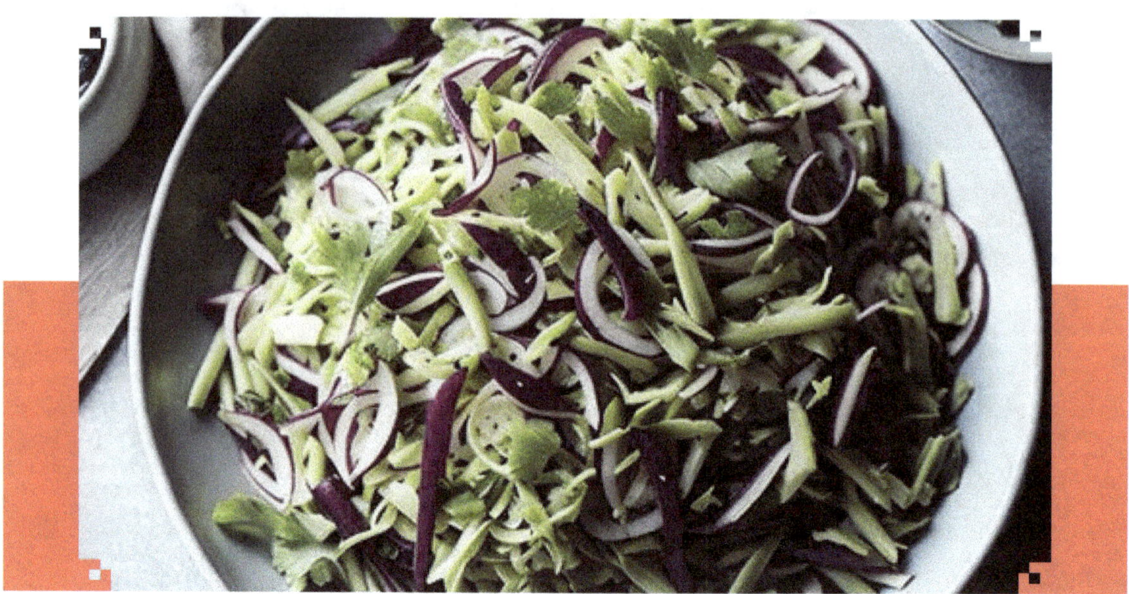

## Coconut Chives Sprouts

**Prep time: 5 minutes |Cook time: 20 minutes |Serves 4**

- 1 pound brussels sprouts, trimmed and halved
- salt and black pepper to the taste
- 2 tablespoons ghee, melted
- ½ cup coconut cream
- 2 tablespoons garlic, minced
- 1 tablespoon chives, chopped

1. In your air fryer, mix the sprouts with the rest of the ingredients except the chives, toss well, introduce in the air fryer and cook them at 370 °F for 20 minutes.
2. Divide the Brussels sprouts between plates, sprinkle the chives on top and serve as a side dish.

### PER SERVING

Calories: 194g| Fat: 6g| Fiber: 2g| Carbs: 4g| Protein: 8 g

## Balsamic Cabbage Mix

**Prep time: 5 minutes |Cook time: 15 minutes |Serves 4**

- 6 cups green cabbage, shredded
- 6 radishes, sliced
- ½ cup celery leaves, chopped
- ¼ cup green onions, chopped
- 2 tablespoons balsamic vinegar
- 1 teaspoon lemon juice
- 3 tablespoons olive oil
- ½ teaspoon hot paprika

1. In your air fryer's pan, combine all the ingredients and toss well.
2. Introduce the pan in the fryer and cook at 380 °F for 15 minutes.
3. Divide between plates and serve as a side dish.

### PER SERVING

Calories: 130g| Fat: 4g| Fiber: 3g| Carbs: 4g| Protein: 7 g

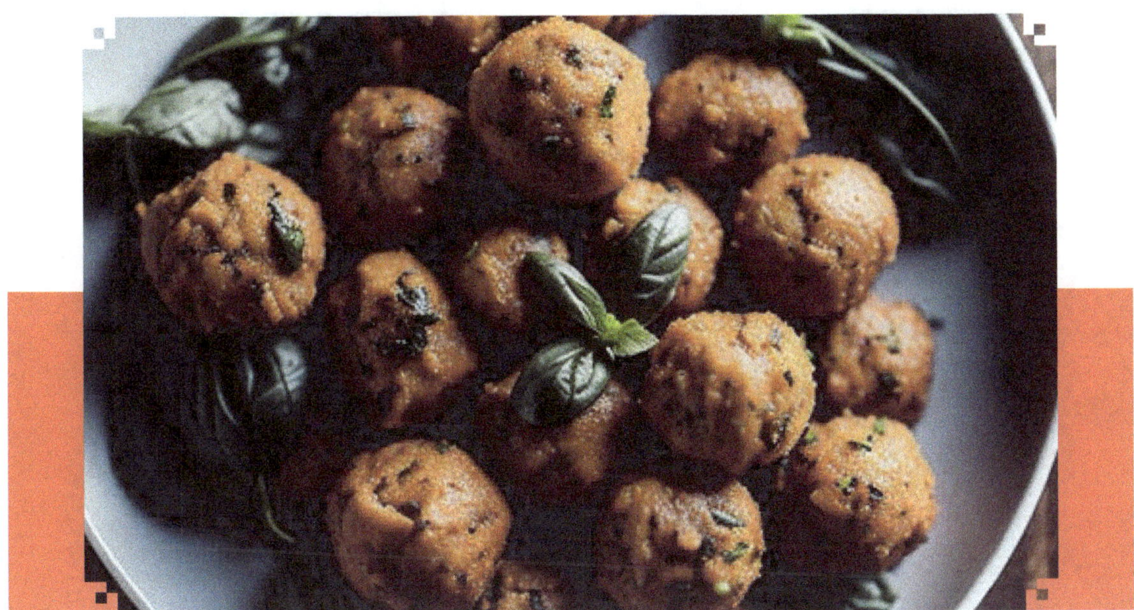

## Garlic Endives and Scallions

**Prep time: 5 minutes |Cook time: 20 minutes |Serves 4**

- 2 scallions, chopped
- 3 garlic cloves, minced
- 1 tablespoon olive oil
- salt and black pepper to the taste
- 1 teaspoon chili sauce
- 4 endives, trimmed and roughly shredded

1. Grease a pan that fits your air fryer with the oil, add all the ingredients, toss, introduce in the air fryer and cook at 370 °F for 20 minutes.
2. Divide everything between plates and serve.

**PER SERVING**

Calories: 184g| Fat: 2g| Fiber: 2g| Carbs: 3g| Protein: 5g

## Seafood Balls

**Prep time: 15 minutes | Cook time: 15 minutes | Serves 4**

- 1-pound salmon fillet, minced
- 1 egg, beaten
- 3 tablespoons coconut, shredded
- ½ cup almond flour
- 1 tablespoon avocado oil
- 1 teaspoon dried basil

1. In the mixing bowl, mix minced salmon fillet, egg, coconut, almond flour, and dried basil.
2. Make the balls from the fish mixture and put them in the air fryer basket.
3. Sprinkle the balls with avocado oil and cook at 365°F for 15 minutes.

**PER SERVING**

Calories: 268 | Fat: 16.4g | Fiber: 2g | Carbs: 3.9g | Protein: 26.6 g

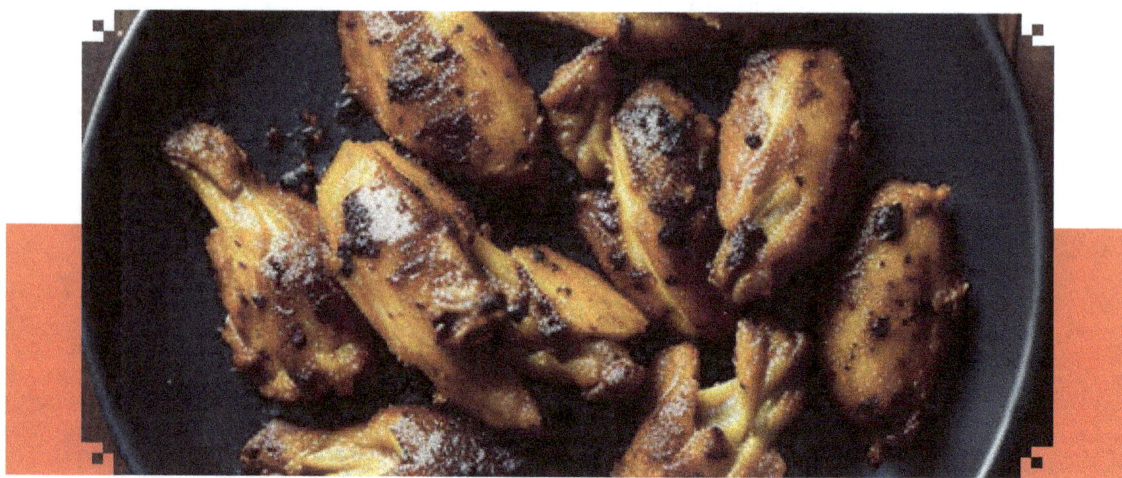

## Italian Cheese Chips

**Prep time: 10 minutes | Cook time: 15 minutes | Serves 4**

- 1 cup Parmesan cheese, shredded
- 1 cup Cheddar cheese, shredded
- 1 teaspoon Italian seasoning
- 1/2 cup marinara sauce

1. Start by preheating your Air Fryer to 350 °F. Place a piece of parchment paper in the cooking basket.
2. Mix the cheese with the Italian seasoning.
3. Add about 1 tablespoon of the cheese mixture (per crisp) to the basket, making sure they are not touching. Bake for 6 minutes or until browned to your liking.
4. Work in batches and place them on a large tray to cool slightly. Serve with the marinara sauce. Bon appétit!

**PER SERVING**

Calories: 231 | Fat: 16.5g | Carbs: 6.4g | Protein: 14g | Fiber: 0.7g

## Dry Rub Chicken Wings

**Prep time: 15 minutes | Cook time: 10 minutes | Serves 4**

- 1 tablespoon paprika
- 1 tablespoon swerve sugar replacement
- ½ teaspoon dried oregano
- ½ teaspoon garlic powder
- ½ teaspoon cayenne
- 1 pound chicken wings, tips removed

1. In a large bowl, combine the paprika, Swerve, oregano, garlic powder, black pepper, and cayenne. Add the coated cover and refrigerate for at least 1 hour or up to 8 hours.
2. Preheat the air fryer to 400°F.
3. Working in batches if necessary, arrange the wings in a single layer in the air fryer basket. crispy and a thermometer inserted into the thickest part registers 165°F.

**PER SERVING**

Calories: 290 | Protein: 27g | Carbs: 1g | Fat: 19g | Fiber: 1g

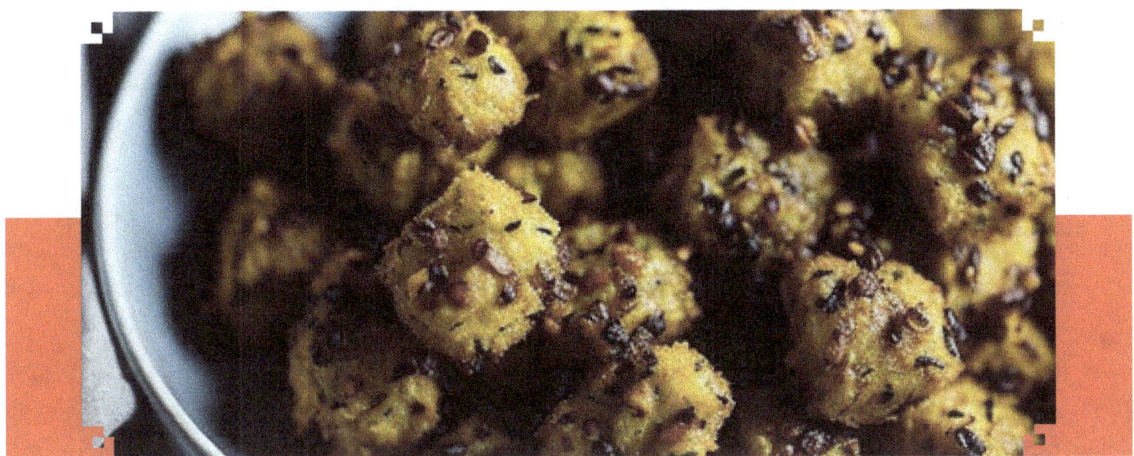

# Bacon and Egg Bites

**Prep time: 15 minutes | Cook time: 10 minutes |
Serves 4**

- 6 ounces (about 9 slices) reduced-sodium bacon
- 2 hard-boiled eggs, chopped
- 2 tablespoons unsalted butter, softened
- 2 tablespoons chopped fresh cilantro
- juice of ½ lime
- salt and freshly ground black pepper

1. Arrange the bacon in a single layer in the air fryer basket Finely chop the bacon and set aside in a small, shallow bowl.
2. Add the reserved bacon grease to the egg mixture and stir gently until or until the mixture is firm.
3. Divide the mixture into 12 equal portions and shape into balls. Roll the balls in the chopped bacon bits until completely coated.

**PER SERVING**

Calories: 330 | Protein: 10g | Carbs: 2g | Fat: 31g | Fiber: 0g

# Chili Zucchini Tots

**Prep time: 10 minutes | Cook time: 12 minutes |
Serves 4**

- 3 zucchinis, grated
- ½ cup coconut flour
- 2 eggs, beaten
- 1 teaspoon chili flakes
- 1 teaspoon salt
- 1 teaspoon avocado oil

1. In the bowl mix up grated carrot, salt, ground cumin, zucchini, Provolone cheese, chili flakes, egg, and coconut flour. Stir the mass with the help of the spoon and make the small balls.
2. Then line the air fryer basket with baking paper and sprinkle it with sunflower oil. Put the zucchini balls in the air fryer basket and cook them for 12 minutes at 375°F.
3. Shake the balls every 2 minutes to avoid burning.

**PER SERVING**

Calories: 122 | Fat: 7.4g | Fiber: 3.7g | Carbs: 7.3g | Protein: 7.2 g

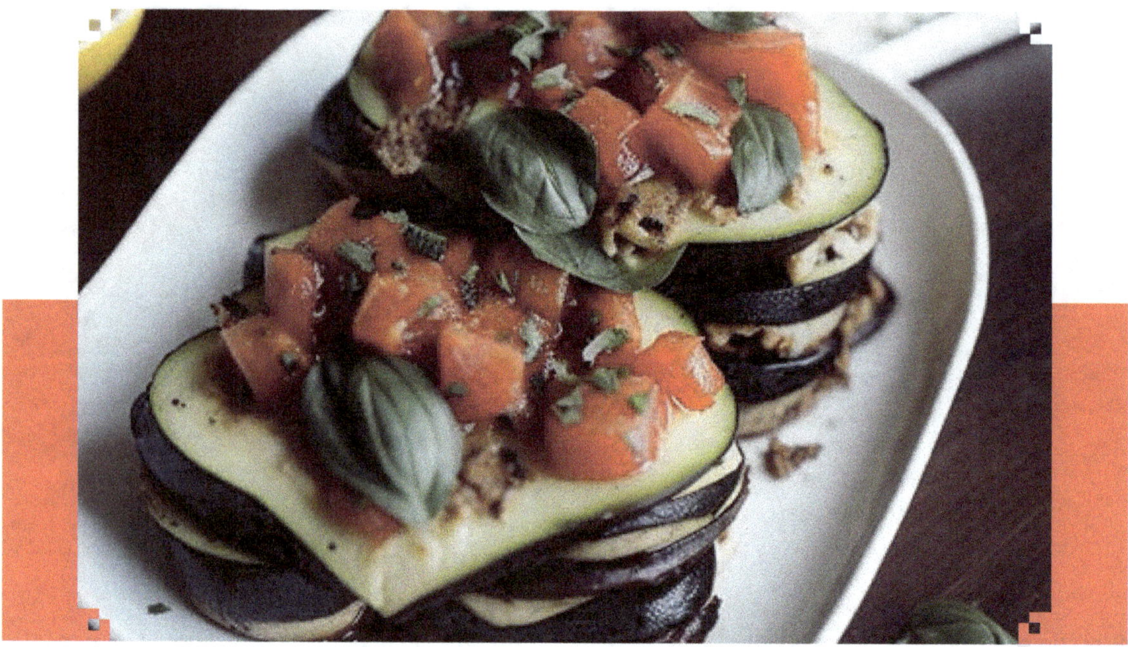

# Savory Herb Cloud Eggs

**Prep time: 5 minutes | Cook time: 8 minutes | Serves 2**

- 2 large eggs, whites and yolks separated
- ¼ teaspoon salt
- ¼ teaspoon dried oregano
- 2 tablespoons chopped fresh chives
- 2 teaspoons salted butter, melted

1. In a large bowl, whip egg whites until stiff peaks form, about 3 minutes. Place 1 whole egg yolk in center of each ramekin and drizzle with butter.
2. Place ramekins into air fryer basket. Egg whites will be fluffy and browned when done. Serve warm.

**PER SERVING**

Calories: 105 | Protein: 6g | Fiber: 0g | Carbs: 1g | Fat: 8g

# Italian Eggplant Bites

**Prep time: 10 minutes |Cook time: 10 minutes |Serves 5**

- 2 medium eggplants, trimmed
- 1 tomato
- 1 teaspoon italian seasonings
- 1 teaspoon avocado oil
- 3 oz parmesan, sliced

1. Slice the eggplants on 5 slices. Then thinly slice the tomato on 5 slices.
2. Place the eggplants in the air fryer in every side at 400°F.
3. After this, top the sliced eggplants then top the eggplants with Parmesan.
4. Cook the meal for 4 minutes at 400°F.

**PER SERVING**

Calories: 116g| Fat: 4.5g| Fiber: 7.9g| Carbs: 14.1g| Protein: 7.7g

# Chapter 9

## Vegan & Vegetarian

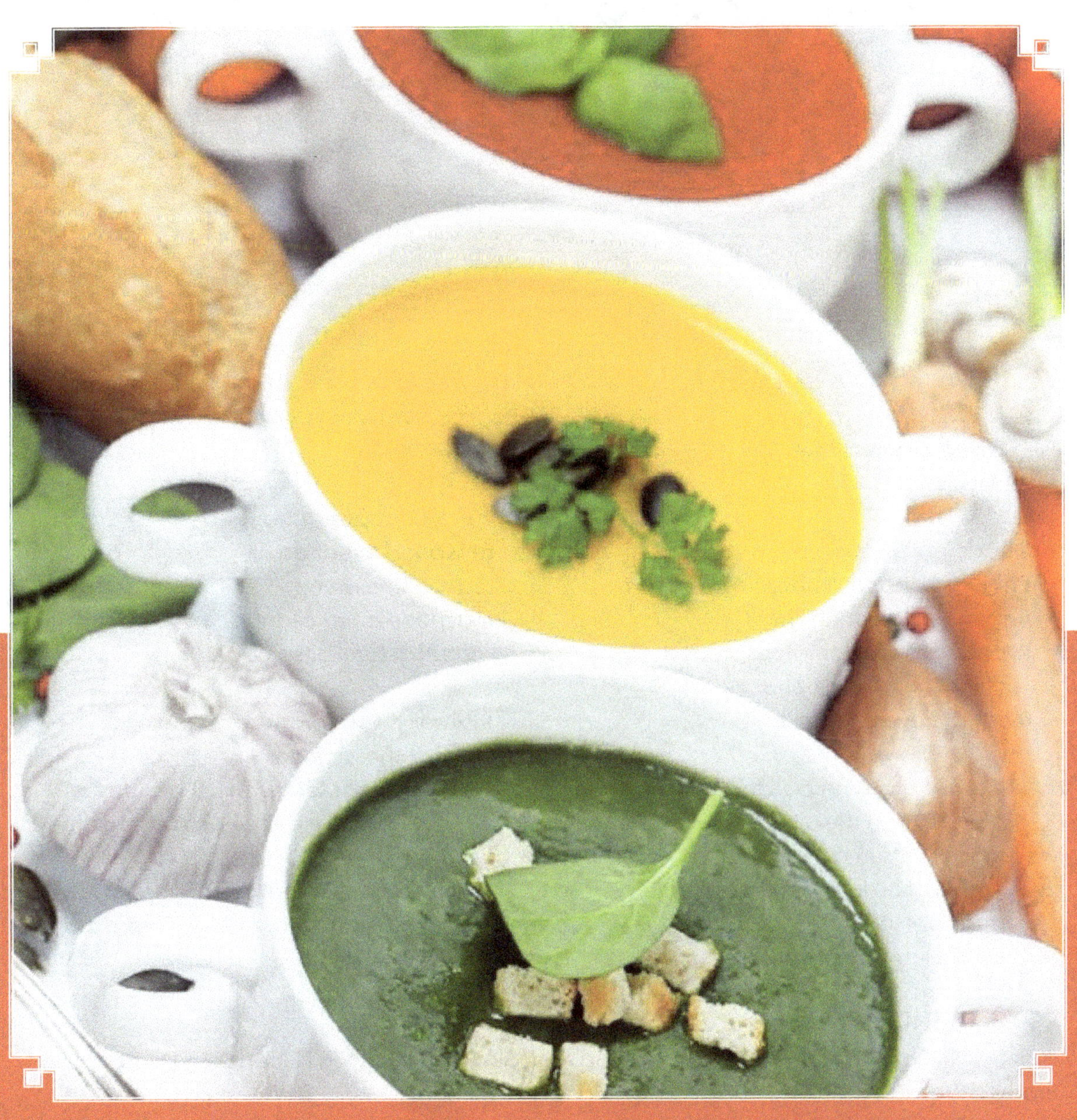

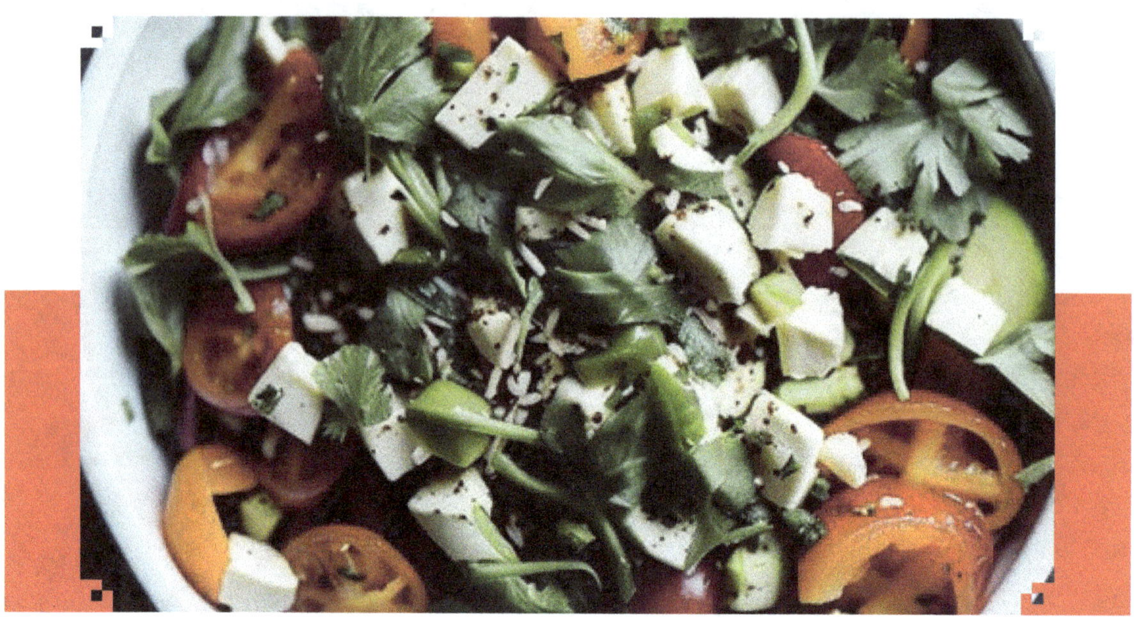

## Tomato and Eggplant Casserole

**Prep time: 5 minutes |Cook time: 20 minutes |Serves 4**

- 2 eggplants, cubed
- 1 hot chili pepper, chopped
- 4 spring onions, chopped
- ½ pound cherry tomatoes, cubed
- ½ cup cilantro, chopped
- 4 garlic cloves, minced

1. Grease a baking pan that fits the air fryer with the oil, and mix all the ingredients in the pan.
2. Put the pan in the preheated air fryer and cook at 380 °F for 20 minutes, divide into bowls and serve for lunch.

**PER SERVING**

Calories: 232g| Fat: 12g| Fiber: 3g| Carbs: 5g| Protein: 10g

## Baked Bell Peppers Salad

**Prep time: 5 minutes | Cook time: 10 minutes | Serves 4**

- 1 cup bell pepper, chopped
- 1 teaspoon avocado oil
- 1 teaspoon olive oil
- 1 teaspoon dried cilantro
- ½ cup Mozzarella, shredded

1. Mix bell pepper with avocado oil and put it in the air fryer.
2. Cook the vegetables for 10 minutes at 385°F. Shake the bell peppers from time to time.
3. Then mix cooked bell peppers with olive oil, cilantro, and Mozzarella. Shake the cooked salad.

**PER SERVING**

Calories: 31 | Fat: 2g | Fiber: 0.5g | Carbs: 2.5g | Protein: 1.3

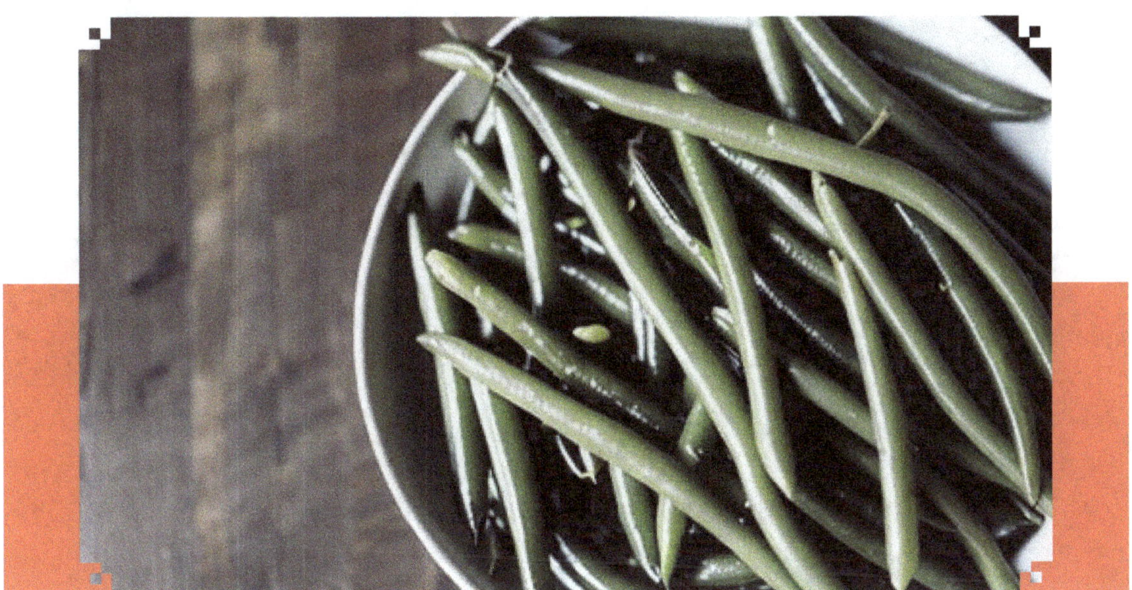

# Crispy Leek Strips

**Prep time: 10 minutes | Cook time: 52 minutes | Serves 6**

- 1/2 teaspoon porcini powder
- 1 cup almond flour
- 1/2 cup coconut flour
- 2 large-sized dishes with ice water
- 2 teaspoons onion powder
- Fine sea salt and cayenne pepper, to taste

1. Allow the leeks to soak in ice water for about 25 minutes; drain well.
2. Drizzle vegetable oil over the seasoned leeks. Air fry at 390 °F for about 18 minutes; turn them halfway through the cooking time.
3. Serve with homemade mayonnaise or any other sauce for dipping. Enjoy!

**PER SERVING**

Calories: 589 | Fat: 47g | Carbs: 6.3g | Protein: 33.1g | Fiber: 2g

# Crispy Green Beans

**Prep time: 5 minutes | Cook time: 8 minutes | Serves 4**

- 2 teaspoons olive oil
- ½ pound fresh green beans, ends trimmed
- ¼ teaspoon salt
- ¼ teaspoon ground black pepper

1. In a large bowl, drizzle olive oil over green beans and sprinkle with salt and pepper.
2. Place green beans into ungreased air fryer basket. Adjust the temperature to 350°F and set the timer for 8 minutes, shaking the basket two times during cooking. Green beans will be dark golden and crispy at the edges when done. Serve warm.

**PER SERVING**

Calories: 37 | Protein: 1g | Fiber: 2g | Carbs: 2g | Fat: 2g

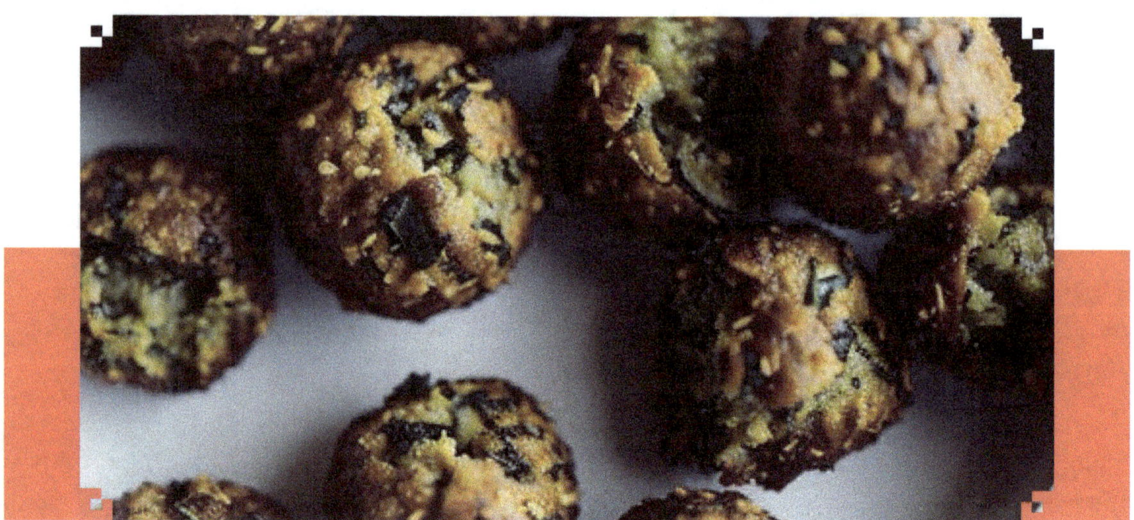

## Dijon Roast Cabbage

**Prep time: 10 minutes | Cook time: 10 minutes | Serves 4**

- 1 small head cabbage, cored and sliced into 1"-thick slices
- 2 tablespoons olive oil, divided
- ½ teaspoon salt
- 1 tablespoon dijon mustard
- 1 teaspoon apple cider vinegar
- 1 teaspoon granular erythritol

1. Drizzle each cabbage slice with 1 tablespoon olive oil, then sprinkle with salt. Adjust the temperature to 350°F and set the timer for 10 minutes. Cabbage will be tender and edges will begin to brown when done.
2. In a small bowl, whisk remaining. Drizzle over cabbage in a large serving dish. Serve warm.

**PER SERVING**

Calories: 111 | Protein: 3g | Fiber: 4g | Carbs: 7g | Fat: 7g

## Thai Zucchini Balls

**Prep time: 10 minutes | Cook time: 30 minutes | Serves 4**

- 1 pound zucchini, grated
- 1 tablespoon orange juice
- 1/2 teaspoon ground cinnamon
- 1/4 teaspoon ground cloves
- 1/2 cup almond meal
- 1 teaspoon baking powder
- 1 cup coconut flakes

1. In a mixing bowl, thoroughly combine all ingredients, except for coconut flakes.
2. Roll the balls in the coconut flakes.
3. Bake in the preheated Air Fryer at 360 °F for 15 minutes or until thoroughly cooked and crispy.
4. Repeat the process until you run out of ingredients. Bon appétit!

**PER SERVING**

Calories: 166 | Fat: 13.1g | Carbs: 9.6g | Protein: 6.2g | Fiber: 4.7g

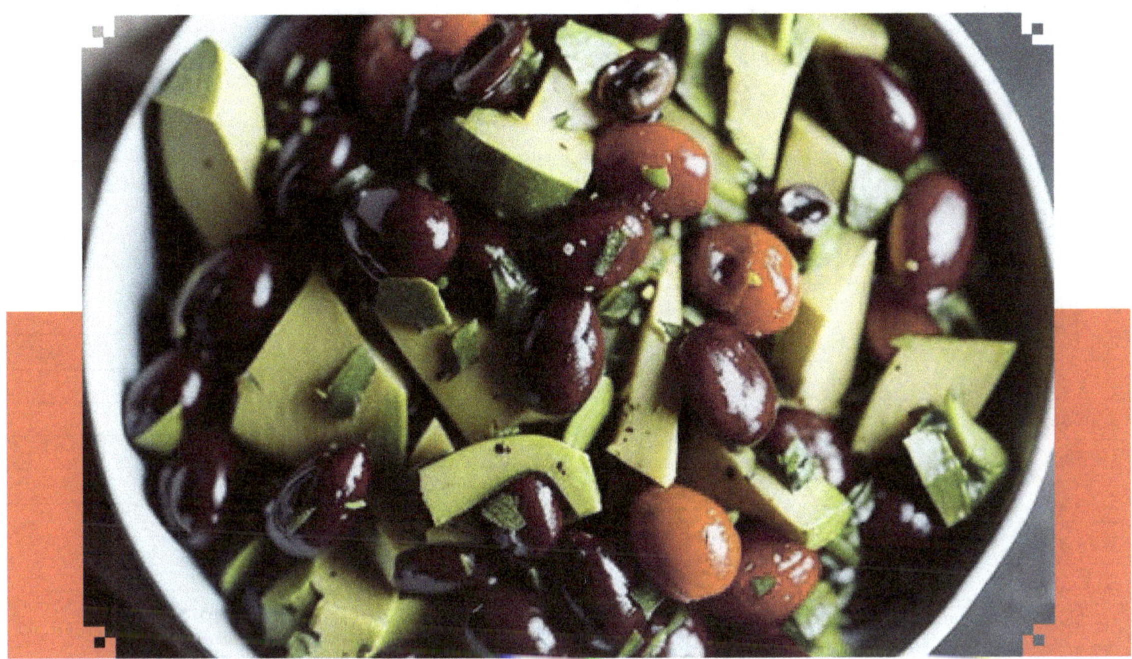

## Crispy Tofu

**Prep time: 15 minutes | Cook time: 10 minutes |**
**Serves 4**

- 1 (16-ounce) block extra-firm tofu
- 2 tablespoons reduced-sodium soy sauce
- 1 tablespoon olive oil
- 1 tablespoon chili-garlic sauce
- 1 scallion, thinly sliced

1. Press the tofu for at least 15 minutes setting a heavy pan on top so that the moisture drains.
2. Preheat the air fryer to 400°F.
3. Arrange the tofu in a single layer in the sprinkled with the sesame seeds and sliced scallion.

**PER SERVING**

Calories: 180 | Protein: 11g | Carbs: 5g | Fat: 13g | Fiber: 1g

## Spicy Olives and Tomato Mix

**Prep time: 5 minutes |Cook time: 15 minutes**
**|Serves 4**

- 2 cups kalamata olives, pitted
- 2 small avocados, pitted, peeled and sliced
- ¼ cup cherry tomatoes, halved
- juice of 1 lime
- 1 tablespoon coconut oil, melted

1. In a pan that fits the air fryer, combine the olives with the other ingredients, toss, put the pan in your air fryer and cook at 370 °F for 15 minutes.
2. Divide the mix between plates and serve.

**PER SERVING**

Calories: 153g| Fat: 3g| Fiber: 3g| Carbs: 4g| Protein: 6g

# Appendix 1 Measurement Conversion Chart

## Volume Equivalents (Dry)

| US STANDARD | METRIC (APPROXIMATE) |
| --- | --- |
| 1/8 teaspoon | 0.5 mL |
| 1/4 teaspoon | 1 mL |
| 1/2 teaspoon | 2 mL |
| 3/4 teaspoon | 4 mL |
| 1 teaspoon | 5 mL |
| 1 tablespoon | 15 mL |
| 1/4 cup | 59 mL |
| 1/2 cup | 118 mL |
| 3/4 cup | 177 mL |
| 1 cup | 235 mL |
| 2 cups | 475 mL |
| 3 cups | 700 mL |
| 4 cups | 1 L |

## Volume Equivalents (Liquid)

| US STANDARD | US STANDARD (OUNCES) | METRIC (APPROXIMATE) |
| --- | --- | --- |
| 2 tablespoons | 1 fl.oz. | 30 mL |
| 1/4 cup | 2 fl.oz. | 60 mL |
| 1/2 cup | 4 fl.oz. | 120 mL |
| 1 cup | 8 fl.oz. | 240 mL |
| 1 1/2 cup | 12 fl.oz. | 355 mL |
| 2 cups or 1 pint | 16 fl.oz. | 475 mL |
| 4 cups or 1 quart | 32 fl.oz. | 1 L |
| 1 gallon | 128 fl.oz. | 4 L |

## Weight Equivalents

| US STANDARD | METRIC (APPROXIMATE) |
| --- | --- |
| 1 ounce | 28 g |
| 2 ounces | 57 g |
| 5 ounces | 142 g |
| 10 ounces | 284 g |
| 15 ounces | 425 g |
| 16 ounces (1 pound) | 455 g |
| 1.5 pounds | 680 g |
| 2 pounds | 907 g |

## Temperatures Equivalents

| FAHRENHEIT(F) | CELSIUS(C) APPROXIMATE) |
| --- | --- |
| 225 °F | 107 °C |
| 250 °F | 120 ° °C |
| 275 °F | 135 °C |
| 300 °F | 150 °C |
| 325 °F | 160 °C |
| 350 °F | 180 °C |
| 375 °F | 190 °C |
| 400 °F | 205 °C |
| 425 °F | 220 °C |
| 450 °F | 235 °C |
| 475 °F | 245 °C |
| 500 °F | 260 °C |

# Appendix 2 The Dirty Dozen and Clean Fifteen

The Environmental Working Group (EWG) is a nonprofit, nonpartisan organization dedicated to protecting human health and the environment Its mission is to empower people to live healthier lives in a healthier environment. This organization publishes an annual list of the twelve kinds of produce, in sequence, that have the highest amount of pesticide residue-the Dirty Dozen-as well as a list of the fifteen kinds ofproduce that have the least amount of pesticide residue-the Clean Fifteen.

| THE DIRTY DOZEN | |
| --- | --- |
| The 2016 Dirty Dozen includes the following produce. These are considered among the year's most Important produce to buy organic: | |
| Strawberries | Spinach |
| Apples | Tomatoes |
| Nectarines | Bell peppers |
| Peaches | Cherry tomatoes |
| Celery | Cucumbers |
| Grapes | Kale/collard greens |
| Cherries | Hot peppers |
| The Dirty Dozen list contains two additional itemskale/collard greens and hot peppers-because they tend to contain trace levels of highly hazardous pesticides. | |

| THE CLEAN FIFTEEN | |
| --- | --- |
| The least critical to buy organically are the Clean Fifteen list. The following are on the 2016 list: | |
| Avocados | Papayas |
| Corn | Kiw |
| Pineapples | Eggplant |
| Cabbage | Honeydew |
| Sweet peas | Grapefruit |
| Onions | Cantaloupe |
| Asparagus | Cauliflower |
| Mangos | |
| Some of the sweet corn sold in the United States are made from genetically engineered (GE) seedstock. Buy organic varieties of these crops to avoid GE produce. | |

# Appendix 3: Keto-Friendly Foods and Foods to Avoid

## KETO FOODS TO ENJOY

### HIGH FAT / LOW CARB (BASED ON NET CARBS)

### MEATS & SEAFOOD

- Beef (ground beef, steak, etc.)
- Chicken
- Crab
- Crawfish
- Duck
- Fish
- Goose
- Lamb
- Lobster
- Mussels
- Octopus
- Pork (pork chops, bacon, etc.)
- Quail
- Sausage (without fillers)
- Scallops
- Shrimp
- Veal
- Venison

### DAIRY

- Blue cheese dressing
- Burrata cheese
- Cottage cheese
- Cream cheese
- Eggs
- Greek yogurt (full-fat)
- Grilling cheese
- Halloumi cheese
- Heavy (whipping) cream
- Kefalotyri cheese
- Mozzarella cheese
- Provolone cheese
- Queso blanco
- Ranch dressing
- Ricotta cheese
- Unsweetened almond milk
- Unsweetened coconut milk

### VEGETABLES

- Alfalfa sprouts
- Asparagus
- Avocados
- Bell peppers
- Broccoli
- Cabbage
- Carrots (in moderation)
- Cauliflower
- Celery
- Chicory
- Coconut
- Cucumbers
- Garlic (in moderation)
- Green beans
- Herbs
- Jicama
- Lemons
- Limes
- Mushrooms
- Okra
- Olives
- Onions (in moderation)
- Pickles
- Pumpkin
- Radishes
- Salad greens
- Scallions
- Spaghetti squash (in moderation)
- Tomatoes (in moderation)
- Zucchini

### NUTS & SEEDS

- Almonds
- Brazil nuts
- Chia seeds
- Flaxseeds
- Hazelnuts
- Macadamia nuts
- Peanuts (in moderation)
- Pecans
- Pine nuts
- Pumpkin seeds
- Sacha inchi seeds
- Sesame seeds
- Walnuts

### FRUITS

- Blackberries
- Blueberries
- Cranberries
- Raspberries
- Strawberries

# KETO FOODS TO AVOID

## LOW FAT / HIGH CARB (BASED ON NET CARBS)

### MEATS & MEAT ALTERNATIVES

- Deli meat (some, not all)
- Hot dogs (with fillers)
- Sausage (with fillers)
- Seitan
- Tofu

### DAIRY

- Almond milk (sweetened)
- Coconut milk (sweetened)
- Milk
- Soy milk (regular)
- Yogurt (regular)

### NUTS & SEEDS

- Cashews
- Chestnuts
- Pistachios

### VEGETABLES

- Artichokes
- Beans (all varieties)
- Burdock root
- Butternut squash
- Chickpeas
- Corn
- Edamame
- Eggplant
- Leeks
- Parsnips
- Plantains
- Potatoes
- Sweet potatoes
- Winter squash
- Oranges
- Yams

### FRUITS &

- Apples
- Apricots
- Bananas
- Boysenberries
- Cantaloupe
- Cherries
- Currants
- Dates
- Elderberries
- Gooseberries
- Grapes
- Honeydew melon
- Huckleberries
- Kiwifruits
- Taro root
- Turnips
- Mangos
- Peaches
- Peas
- Pineapples
- Plums
- Prunes
- Raisins
- Water chestnuts

## KETO COOKING STAPLES

1. Pink Himalayan salt
2. Freshly ground black pepper
3. 3 Ghee (clarified butter, without dairy; buy
4. grass-fed if you can)
5. 4 Olive oil
6. Grass-fed butter

## KETO PERISHABLES

Eggs (pasture-raised, if you can)
2 Avocados
3 Bacon (uncured)
Cream cheese (full-fat; or use a dairy-free alterna- tive)
Sour cream (full-fat; or use a dairy-free alternative)
Heavy whipping cream or coconut milk (full-fat; I buy the coconut milk in a can)
Garlic (fresh or pre-minced in a jar)
Meat (grass-fed, if you can)
10 Greens (spinach, kale, or arugula)

# Appendix 4: Air Fryer Cooking Chart

## Air Fryer Cooking Chart

| Beef | | | | | |
|---|---|---|---|---|---|
| Item | Temp (°F) | Time (mins) | Item | Temp (°F) | Time (mins) |
| Beef Eye Round Roast (4 lbs.) | 400 °F | 45 to 55 | Meatballs (1-inch) | 370 °F | 7 |
| Burger Patty (4 oz.) | 370 °F | 16 to 20 | Meatballs (3-inch) | 380 °F | 10 |
| Filet Mignon (8 oz.) | 400 °F | 18 | Ribeye, bone-in (1-inch, 8 oz) | 400 °F | 10 to 15 |
| Flank Steak (1.5 lbs.) | 400 °F | 12 | Sirloin steaks (1-inch, 12 oz) | 400 °F | 9 to 14 |
| Flank Steak (2 lbs.) | 400 °F | 20 to 28 | | | |

| Chicken | | | | | |
|---|---|---|---|---|---|
| Item | Temp (°F) | Time (mins) | Item | Temp (°F) | Time (mins) |
| Breasts, bone in (1 1/4 lb.) | 370 °F | 25 | Legs, bone-in lb.) | 380 °F | 30 |
| Breasts, boneless (4 oz) | 380 °F | 12 | Thighs, boneless (1 1/2 lb.) | 380 °F | 18 to 20 |
| Drumsticks (2 1/2 lb.) | 370 °F | 20 | Wings (2 lb.) | 400 °F | 12 |
| Game Hen (halved 2 lb.) | 390 °F | 20 | Whole Chicken | 360 °F | 75 |
| Thighs, bone-in (2 lb.) | 380 °F | 22 | Tenders | 360 °F | 8 to 10 |

| Pork & Lamb | | | | | |
| --- | --- | --- | --- | --- | --- |
| Item | Temp (°F) | Time (mins) | Item | Temp (°F) | Time (mins) |
| Bacon (regular) | 400 °F | 5 to 7 | Pork Tenderloin | 370 °F | 15 |
| Bacon (thick cut) | 400 °F | 6 to 10 | Sausages | 380 °F | 15 |
| Pork Loin (2 lb.) | 360 °F | 55 | Lamb Loin Chops (1-inch thick) | 400 °F | 8 to 12 |
| Pork Chops, bone in (1-inch, 6.5 oz) | 400 °F | 12 | Rack of Lamb (1.5 - lb.) | 380 °F | 22 |
| Flank Steak (2 lbs.) | 400 °F | 20 to 28 | | | |

| Fish & Seafood | | | | | |
| --- | --- | --- | --- | --- | --- |
| Item | Temp (°F) | Time (mins) | Item | Temp (°F) | Time (mins) |
| Calamari (8 oz) | 400 °F | 4 | Tuna Steak | 400 °F | 7 to 10 |
| Fish Fillet (1-inch, 8 oz) | 400 °F | 10 | Scallops | 400 °F | 5 to 7 |
| Salmon, fillet (6 oz) | 380 °F | 12 | Shrimp | 400 °F | 5 |
| Swordfish steak | 400 °F | 10 | Sirloin steaks (1-inch, 12 oz) | 400 °F | 9 to 14 |
| Flank Steak (2 lbs.) | 400 °F | 20 to 28 | | | |

**Vegetables**

| INGREDIENT | AMOUNT | PREPARATION | OIL | TEMP | COOK TIME |
|---|---|---|---|---|---|
| Asparagus | 2 bunches | Cut in half, trim stems | 2 Tbsp | 420°F | 12–15 mins |
| Beets | 1 1/2 lbs | Peel, cut in 1/2-inch cubes | 1 Tbsp | 390°F | 28–30 mins |
| Bell peppers (for roasting) | 4 peppers | Cut in quarters, remove seeds | 1 Tbsp | 400°F | 15–20 mins |
| Broccoli | 1 large head | Cut in 1-2-inch florets | 1 Tbsp | 400°F | 15–20 mins |
| Brussels sprouts | 1 lb | Cut in half, remove stems | 1 Tbsp | 425°F | 15–20 mins |
| Carrots | 1 lb | Peel, cut in 1/4-inch rounds | 1 Tbsp | 425°F | 10–15 mins |
| Cauliflower | 1 head | Cut in 1-2-inch florets | 2 Tbsp | 400°F | 20–22 mins |
| Corn on the cob | 7 ears | Whole ears, remove husks | 1 Tbps | 400°F | 14–17 mins |
| Green beans | 1 bag (12 oz) | Trim | 1 Tbps | 420°F | 18–20 mins |
| Kale (for chips) | 4 OZ | Tear into pieces, remove stems | None | 325°F | 5–8 mins |
| Mushrooms | 16 OZ | Rinse, slice thinly | 1 Tbps | 390°F | 25–30 mins |
| Potatoes, russet | 1 1/2 lbs | Cut in 1-inch wedges | 1 Tbps | 390°F | 25–30 mins |
| Potatoes, russet | 1 lb | Hand-cut fries, soak 30 mins in cold water, then pat dry | 1/2 –3 Tbps | 400°F | 25–28 mins |
| Potatoes, sweet | 1 lb | Hand-cut fries, soak 30 mins in cold water, then pat dry | 1 Tbps | 400°F | 25–28 mins |
| Zucchini | 1 lb | Cut in eighths lengthwise, then cut in half | 1 Tbps | 400°F | 15–20 mins |

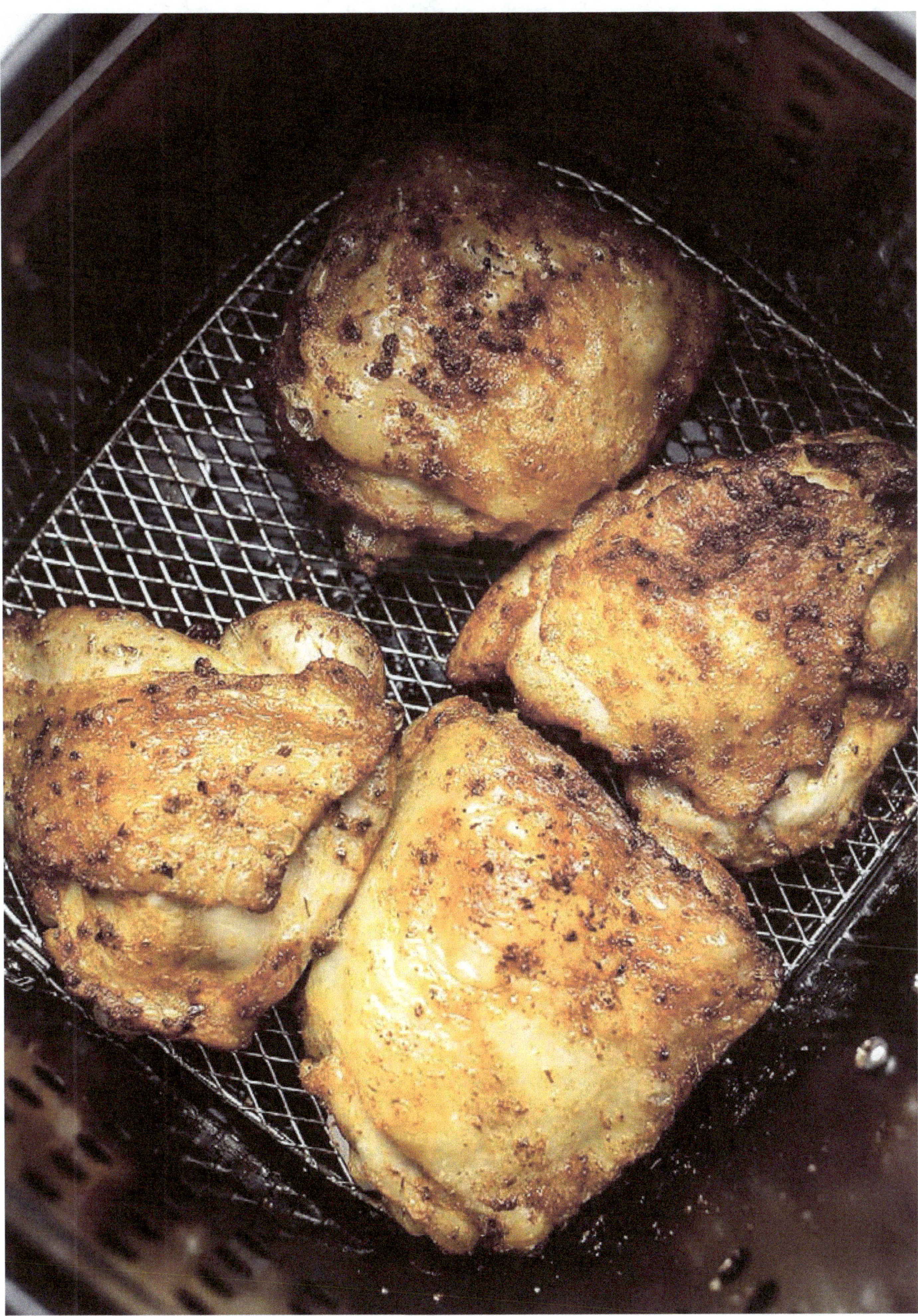

# Appendix 5 Index

**Hey there!**

Wow, can you believe we've reached the end of this culinary journey together? I'm truly thrilled and filled with joy as I think back on all the recipes we've shared and the flavors we've discovered. This experience, blending a bit of tradition with our own unique twists, has been a journey of love for good food. And knowing you've been out there, giving these dishes a try, has made this adventure incredibly special to me.

Even though we're turning the last page of this book, I hope our conversation about all things delicious doesn't have to end. I cherish your thoughts, your experiments, and yes, even those moments when things didn't go as planned. Every piece of feedback you share is invaluable, helping to enrich this experience for us all.

I'd be so grateful if you could take a moment to share your thoughts with me, be it through a review on Amazon or any other place you feel comfortable expressing yourself online. Whether it's praise, constructive criticism, or even an idea for how we might do things differently in the future, your input is what truly makes this journey meaningful.

This book is a piece of my heart, offered to you with all the love and enthusiasm I have for cooking. But it's your engagement and your words that elevate it to something truly extraordinary.

Thank you from the bottom of my heart for being such an integral part of this culinary adventure. Your openness to trying new things and sharing your experiences has been the greatest gift.

**Catch you later,**

**Felicia W. McCloud**

Printed in the USA
CPSIA information can be obtained
at www.ICGtesting.com
CBHW081558060724
11233CB00019B/1580